THE GLUTEN-FREE GOOD HEALTH COOKBOOK

ANNALISE G. ROBERTS AND CLAUDIA PILLOW, PhD

THE GLUTEN-FREE GOOD HEALTH COOKBOOK

The Delicious Way to Strengthen Your Immune System and Neutralize Inflammation

ANNALISE G. ROBERTS AND CLAUDIA PILLOW, PhD

SURREY BOOKS

AGATE

CHICAGO

Layout and design by Brandtner Design.

Printed in the United States of America.

Library of Congress Cataloging-in-Publication Data

Roberts, Annalise G.
 The gluten-free good health cookbook : the delicious way to strengthen your immune system and neutralize inflammation / Annalise G. Roberts and Claudia Pillow.
     p. cm.
 Summary: "A guide, with recipes, to strengthening the immune system, preventing disease, and losing weight though healthful, gluten-free eating"--Provided by publisher.
 Includes bibliographical references and index.
 ISBN-13: 978-1-57284-105-5 (pbk.)
 ISBN-10: 1-57284-105-2 (pbk.)
 1. Gluten-free diet--Recipes. I. Pillow, Claudia. II. Title.
 RM237.86.R584 2010
 641.5'638--dc22
                        2009042437

10 9 8 7 6 5 4 3

Surrey Books is an imprint of Agate Publishing. Agate books are available in bulk at discount prices. Single copies are available prepaid direct from the publisher. For more information visit agatepublishing.com.

We would like to thank all our family and friends, who have taught, challenged, inspired, supported, and ate with us along our culinary journey.

Thank you, Herb and Ev, for an early introduction to the glorious world of food and the pleasures of eating.

Thanks to our little brother Donald, for being a faithful customer at the Little House on the Hill, and to our sister Suzanne, for always being on the cutting edge of the next food trend and forcing us to stay current.

Thanks to Tim, Monica, and Cory for their unconditional love and their never-ending enthusiasm for the next meal.

Thanks to Conrad, Alexander and Bradford, for their love and encouragement, and for always being there to taste and comment on our creations.

Thanks to Douglas Seibold, president and publisher of Agate Publishing, for giving us the opportunity to write this cookbook and expand our world.

Thanks to Perrin Davis, senior vice president of editorial services of Agate Publishing, for seeing it through to the happy end.

TABLE OF CONTENTS

FOREWORD

APPROXIMATELY 1 PERCENT OF THE POPULATION suffers from celiac disease, the form of gluten intolerance that is best understood by most medical professionals. This amounts to about 3 million Americans. Although the medical community as a whole still has a long way to go in recognizing the wide range of symptoms that can be associated with celiac disease, the illness only afflicts a small portion of those who are gluten intolerant. Celiac disease, a highly specific type of damage that occurs in the small intestine, is only one symptom that can result from gluten intolerance. It's believed that as many as 30 million people suffer from gluten intolerance in the United States alone.

Gluten intolerance is certainly a fundamental trigger of many common health problems in this country. Those who have been diagnosed with gluten intolerance or who have figured out for themselves that they are gluten intolerant already understand the significance of this problem and the dramatic impact avoiding gluten can have on their health. I wrote the book *Healthier Without Wheat* to help people discover and understand gluten intolerance and learn how to test themselves for it. Unfortunately, the problem of gluten intolerance is still underestimated by the medical community, and it will be a long time before most people who actually are intolerant are diagnosed.

However, discovering that you are gluten intolerant is just the beginning of your journey. Once you do, you have to learn how to avoid gluten, of course—but just avoiding gluten doesn't necessarily mean that you have healthy eating habits. I've met many people who don't consume gluten but still manage to have gluten-free junk food diets. Many companies are making it easy to do this by creating highly processed and refined gluten-free foods. Yes, if you have a gluten intolerance, avoiding gluten is a major improvement, but it's still a long way from finding a diet that will optimize your health. It will also keep you from fully understanding the impact food has on your life.

For this reason, it's a wonderful change of pace to read a book like *The Gluten-Free Good Health Cookbook*. This cookbook is not just about eating gluten free. It's about reestablishing a healthy relationship with food. Over time, the idea of healthy eating has grown complicated, but it doesn't need to be that way. It's really quite simple, but sometimes we lose our way and need someone to help put us back on track. We need to be reminded exactly what it means to eat real food, healthy food.

That's just what Claudia Pillow and Annalise Roberts do in this valuable and insightful book. Claudia and Annalise provide a number of tools and guidelines to help you understand how to eat healthier and achieve better health. *The Gluten-Free Good Health Cookbook* is a very practical and thorough book that's also alive with an appreciation for whole foods and a well roundedness not found in many other gluten-free cookbooks.

Having had the good fortune of joining Claudia and her family for a home-cooked meal, I can tell you firsthand that she knows how to prepare a very tasty and satisfying meal. There is an honest simplicity to her cooking that brings out her love and understanding of food, flavors, and aromas. And when you enjoy the recipes Claudia and Annalise have created for this book, you'll see that they're healthy and nourishing for both body and soul.

I encourage you to learn and apply the techniques and guidance found in this book. If you do, you'll be richly rewarded at your next meal and for the rest of your life.

—Stephen Wangen, MD
www.HealthierWithoutWheat.com

INTRODUCTION

I HAVE BEEN NEUTRALIZED for several years now. The transformation began after my sister, Annalise Roberts, was diagnosed with celiac disease, and I wanted to support her in her quest for delicious gluten-free food. Together we converted favorite recipes to be gluten free and created new recipes as we cooked and baked our way through the seasons.

And then we took it one step further. Annalise dedicated herself to developing the best gluten-free baking recipes to share with the world. She has been so successful that her recipes were featured in *Gourmet* magazine, and she now has two gluten-free baking cookbooks: *Gluten-Free Baking Classics* and *Gluten-Free Baking Classics for the Bread Machine*. I took another path. I wanted to understand why gluten makes so many people sick in so many different ways. My research led me to a PhD in health studies with a focus on celiac disease. And from my studies, the idea for the *Gluten-Free Good Health Cookbook* was born.

I began teaching gluten-free cooking and nutrition classes in 2005, but I did not decide to go gluten free at that time because I did not suffer from celiac disease. After conducting several classes, however, I felt like a hypocrite and decided to dedicate myself to the diet for two months. Well, I really did feel better. The swelling in my finger and toe joints subsided, my weight stabilized without dieting, and, most importantly, I felt energized. Yes, I missed bagels, pizza, and other gluten-filled favorites, but after two weeks the cravings went away. I further fine-tuned my diet by drinking lemon water in the morning to detoxify, replacing diet soda with green tea, reducing refined sugars, and balancing my intake of vegetables and fruits with protein and carbohydrates. These changes led me to better health, my ideal weight, and less frequent visits to my doctor. That's good medicine, and it's our prescription for you. We want to help you be healthy and neutralized.

When reflecting back on my teaching and research, the most startling and unexpected discovery was the sheer number of people who had constant gastrointestinal problems (especially diarrhea and constipation), arthritis and joint pain, thyroid issues, body aches, and depression. The second unexpected finding was that so few people equated their physical conditions with reactions to the food they ate. Most people rarely spoke about their disorders and discomfort to others, including loved ones. When they did discuss their health issues, they justified their conditions by saying they've got a fast metabolism, they're stressed, they don't get enough sleep, they need to exercise more, or they eat a lot of "bad food" because they eat most of their meals away from home. Diarrhea is not normal and neither is constipation. They are both symptoms of intestinal disorders and diseases. If your dog has diarrhea, the first thing you do is change its diet. Why don't we do that for ourselves?

The medical profession has reinforced a basic flaw in our thinking—that we treat symptoms and not the underlying cause of disease. For example, if you have an upset stomach you are told to take medication to make you feel better rather than think about whether you might have eaten something that made you feel bad. If you have joint swelling, the doctor prescribes anti-inflammatory drugs rather than discussing eating a diet full of anti-inflammatory foods. This thinking needs to change. One of my friends has a teenage son who was diagnosed with colitis, an acute inflammation of the membrane lining the colon in the large intestine. No theories about the causes of colitis have been proven, but medical researchers think the body's immune system reacts to a virus or bacteria by causing ongoing inflammation in the intestinal wall. Some doctors think the immune system's reaction may be a result, not the cause, of the disease. Instead of trying to uncover the underlying cause of the disease, our friend's gastroenterologist wants to remove part of her 16-year-old son's colon. The doctor has repeatedly told her that colitis is not caused by a food allergy or sensitivity. Yet 50 percent of the immune system surrounds the digestive tract, and a healthy gut is essential for a healthy immune system.

Eating foods that trigger the immune system (such as any of the eight top allergens: peanuts, tree nuts, milk, eggs, soybeans, fish, shellfish, and wheat) causes inflammation. Chronic inflammation leads to chronic disease. Colitis is a chronic disease of chronic inflammation. How is colitis not affected by the food we eat? Rather than recommend a change in diet to reduce an inflammatory immune response, the doctor recommended drugs and surgery.

Food sensitivities, including intolerances and allergies, result in negative physiologic reactions. These reactions serve as warning signs that the immune system is challenged. Our bodies are saying "stop," but we just aren't yielding. To reverse this all-out modern-day assault on the immune system we must neutralize inflammation in the body. A strong immune system will lead to better health, physical fitness, weight loss, and mental vigor. Better health will reward you with less physical pain, illness, disease, and mental stress. Instead of being one new drug or miracle cure away from being healthy, slim, and feeling good, let us show you how to take control of your own well-being by eating smart to protect your health.

—*Claudia Pillow, PhD, March 2009*

Understanding the Gluten-Free Good Health Diet

THE *GLUTEN-FREE GOOD HEALTH COOKBOOK* breaks the mold for diet books because it combines basic science and proven medical research with a true love of food and eating—Ph.D. meets Julia Child. The role of diet in the development and treatment of chronic disease is undervalued by the medical profession and the public. Doctors are trained to treat disease with medicine and surgery. The *Gluten-Free Good Health Cookbook* explains how you can take control of your own health in order to strengthen your immune system, prevent disease, and lose weight by eating real food.

The Big Picture

THE FOOD WE EAT is the single most important factor impacting our health and for many of us, our health is not good. We don't make the right food choices. Today, two out of three American adults are overweight, and of those, 35 percent are obese. Most of us eat too much refined wheat and sugar. Fewer than 25 percent of us eat enough fruits and vegetables. Sadly, we pass these bad habits on to our children. One in six kids is overweight, and obesity is the leading health threat to our nation. Obesity is a major contributor to the rising prevalence of chronic disease in this country. *More than 90 million people in the United States live with at least one chronic disease, and the yearly medical care costs are estimated at a mind-boggling $1.5 trillion.* Following is a peek into the window of chronic disease[1]:

- More than 80 million people have cardiovascular disease
- 46 million suffer from arthritis
- 24 million live with type 2 diabetes
- 24 million have allergies, including 8 million children
- 23 million have asthma, including 7 million children
- One in 2 men and 1 in 3 women will develop cancer[2]
- 24 million are affected by autoimmune diseases, such as type 1 diabetes, celiac disease, lupus, and the thyroid disease Hashimoto[3]

We need to take responsibility for our own health. Being in good health improves our quality of life because good health provides the energy to do things we enjoy. Unfortunately, too many people believe it is easier to take medication than to engage in healthy eating and exercise. This unhealthy thinking is reinforced by the medical community, whose goal in caring for patients with chronic conditions is all too often to find treatments (in the form of medicine) that produce fewer side effects. In contrast, what is really needed is prevention-centered healthcare. The significant role of diet in the development and treatment of chronic disease is undervalued in this country. The food we eat is making us very sick, and we are suffering the painful consequences. Our food choices have upset the body's balance. We are anxious, overstimulated, and inflamed. This inflammation weakens the immune system. A weak immune system is the trigger for chronic disease. Strengthening our immune system is the key to health and vitality.

A healthy person has an internal chemistry that is in balance, so his or her immune system is strong. A healthy immune system protects you from chronic inflammation, which causes not only arthritis and body aches but also digestive disorders, allergies, asthma, thyroid problems, and other chronic diseases, such as Alzheimer's disease, cancer, diabetes, and heart disease. You need to eat smart to neutralize the inflammation in your body that causes disease.

Our food choices are upsetting the balance of our body and making us sick with chronic health conditions. These chronic health conditions can appear in any of the body's systems

Cerebral: headaches, migraines, depression, dizziness, sleep disorders, learning disorders, autism, fatigue, irritability, or anxiety

Skeletal: osteoporosis, arthritis, fibromyalgia, joint pain, or short stature

Metabolic and Immune: overweight, obesity, under-weight, anorexia, diabetes, auto-immune diseases (lupus, celiac, Sjogren's, IgA, and multiple sclerosis), mineral deficiencies, or malabsorption

Other body systems: chronic fatigue syndrome, thyroiditis, muscle pain, PMS, fatigue, miscarriage, impotence, numbness, hypoglycemia, or urinary irritation

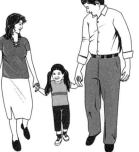

Skin-related: dermatitis, eczema, acne, melanoma, hair loss, hives, or rashes

Cardiovascular: high blood pressure, high cholesterol, hypertension, stroke, nosebleeds, or anemia

Digestive: irritable bowel syndrome, diarrhea, constipation, bloating, gas, colic, heartburn, metabolic syndrome X, diabetes, abdominal pain, vomiting, reflux, gastroenteritis, underweight, malabsorption, celiac disease, colitis, Crohn's disease, leaky gut syndrome, canker sores, enamel defects, or lactose intolerance

Respiratory: hay fever, asthma, allergies, hoarseness, sinus conditions, rhinitis, laryngitis, or recurring ear infections

Modern diet: Refined processed foods ⇨ overreactive immune response ⇨ chronic inflammation ⇨ chronic disease

PHARMA MATTERS

Sixty percent of medical school department heads are paid by pharmaceutical companies as consultants or officers. More than two-thirds of department chairs contend that such close relationships with medical companies have no effect on their professional activities. Third-year medical students receive, on average, one gift or attend one activity sponsored by a drug maker each week.[4]

WHY DO WE NEED TO DEFEND OUR IMMUNE SYSTEM?

Our earliest *Homo sapiens* ancestors from the Middle Paleolithic Era (they appeared about 140,000 years ago) were hunter-gatherers and lived on game animals, seafood, vegetables, fruits, tubers, and nuts. There were no grain crops, such as wheat, and the only sugar they ate was seasonal honey. Early humans benefited from this diet, which was rich in lean protein, complex carbohydrates, vitamins, minerals, omega-3 fatty acids (primarily from fish oil), and other food compounds, such as phytochemicals and flavonoids, that are considered important to health. The Paleolithic diet supplied the proper nutrients to keep the immune system strong enough to fight infectious disease from foreign substances, such as bacteria and viruses. Through the process of evolution, the humans with the strongest immune systems survived, and it left our ancestors hardwired to need a variety of foods for proper nutrition to fight disease.

LEAN + STRONG

EARLY MAN

Modern humans are virtually genetically identical to our ancestors who lived at the end of the Paleolithic Era (10,000 years ago). In fact, the human genome has changed very little since then.[5] The range of foods available to early humans varied widely not only geographically but also seasonally and was far greater than the variety of food we eat today.[6] Now, most of our daily calorie intake comes from just 10 foods: wheat, refined sugar, vegetable oil, refined corn, beef, processed potatoes, iceberg lettuce, canned tomatoes, orange juice, and apples.[5]

This modern diet weakens the immune system, leaving us vulnerable to chronic disease and infections like pneumonia. We need to defend our immune system to stay healthy. Table 1.1 compares the typical diet of the Paleolithic Era with the typical modern diet. We have the same bodies as the people of the Paleolithic Era, but a very different diet.

FAT + WEAK

MODERN MAN

Table 1.1 Typical Diet of Early Humans versus Modern Humans.

EARLY HUMANS (40,000 years ago)	MODERN HUMANS (past 150 years)
Hunter-gatherer lifestyle	Industrial lifestyle
DIET	
65% animal and fish based	35% animal and fish based
35% plant based	65% plant based
No refined wheat or sugar	Lots of refined wheat and sugar
CALORIE INTAKE	
40% carbohydrates (vegetables and fruits)	50% carbohydrates (wheat based)
35% lean protein (wild game)	15% protein (red meat)
25% fats (polyunsaturated)	35% fats (saturated)
OMEGA-6:OMEGA-3 FATTY ACID RATIO	
3:1	12:1
DAILY FIBER INTAKE	
104 grams	15 grams
BEVERAGES	
Water	Soda, coffee, alcohol
PRIMARY CAUSES OF DEATH	
Infections, accidents, complications from childbirth	Chronic diseases (such as heart disease, cancer, diabetes), infections (pneumonia)

WHAT TWO FOODS MAKE UP ALMOST HALF OUR DAILY CALORIES?

Almost half of our calories come from refined wheat and sugars.[7] We consume 34 percent more wheat than we did just 40 years ago, and we eat wheat all day: cereal for breakfast, a sandwich for lunch, cookies and crackers for snacks, and pizza or pasta for dinner. Too much of any one type of food is not a good thing, and all that wheat is poison to the immune system. In fact, celiac disease, a disorder caused by an inappropriate autoimmune reaction to the gluten protein in wheat, is four times (or 400 percent) more common today than it was 50 years ago.[8] Wheat and sugar not only create excess acidity in the body, but they also cause inflammation in the body. The result is an overactive immune system, which increases the risk of autoimmune and chronic diseases, such as cancer, cardiovascular damage, obesity, and type 2 diabetes. As a nation and as individuals, we are not neutralized. Our daily diet must change. For more information, see The Fine Print Appendix A, page 268.

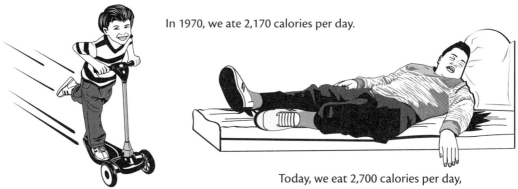

In 1970, we ate 2,170 calories per day.

Today, we eat 2,700 calories per day, or **530 calories** more per day.

DEPRESSION AND DIET

Some form of depression is found in 1 in 10 children and 1 in 14 adults. In the past ten years, use of antidepressant and antianxiety prescription drugs has skyrocketed, but there has been very little discussion about how to prevent depression. Research by the National Institutes of Health[9] has found a direct correlation between lower rates of depression in countries where people typically consume large amounts of fish. Eating fish can prevent depression, slow mental aging, and reduce the risk of suicide.[10] Doesn't it make sense that there could be correlations between high rates of depression and the high consumption of certain foods? In the United States, we eat a lot of wheat and sugar.

BREAKDOWN OF TODAY'S DAILY DIET

825 calories from grains: mostly refined wheat =

10 pieces of bread

490 calories from sugars: mostly high-fructose corn syrup and table sugar =

two sodas and a chocolate bar

475 calories from protein: mostly animal protein =

a 3-ounce serving of both a hamburger and a chicken breast

565 calories from fat: mostly saturated =

5⅔ tablespoons butter

345 calories from other sources: processed potatoes, oranges, and apples =

small order of fries, glass of orange juice, and an apple

50% of daily calories =

wheat (and other grains) and sugar

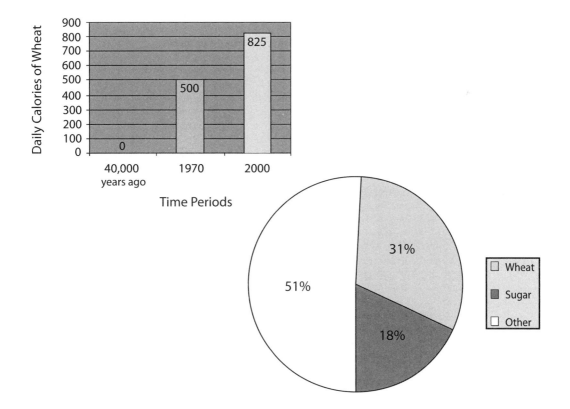

HOW DOES DAILY DIET AFFECT BODY CHEMISTRY?

The most important indicator of body chemistry is pH. All fluids have a pH measure, which is simply the measure of the acidity or alkalinity of a solution. You can measure your body's pH by using pH strips, just like you measure your weight by using a scale. All foods, once eaten and metabolized, combine with the body's fluids and become either acid-forming or alkaline-forming foods. The human body is 80 percent fluid, and we have a genetically encoded acid–alkaline balance requirement very similar to that of our ancestors: blood pH should be 7.4. Early humans ate a diet of more than 50 percent alkaline-forming foods and less than 50 percent acid-forming foods. Modern humans eat a diet of less than 15 percent alkaline-forming foods but more than 85 percent acid-forming foods. Today's diet makes people acidic and does not support the body's natural pH balance. Following are the balanced pH levels of bodily fluids:

- **Blood pH** = 7.4
- **Urine pH** = 6.5 to 7.25
- **Saliva pH** = 6.5 to 7.5

Generally, alkaline-forming foods include most fruits and vegetables, peas, light-colored beans, lentils, spices, herbs and seasonings, green tea, and nuts and seeds. Acid-forming foods include high-protein foods (such as meat, poultry, fish, and eggs), nearly all grains (includ-

We Need to Eat More Alkaline-Forming Foods

These are alkaline-forming (+) food groups that have a pH ≥ 7
Alkaline-forming foods neutralize inflammation

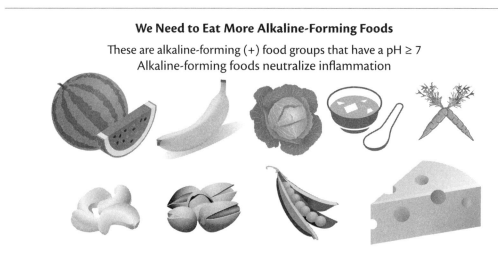

These are acid-neutralizing minerals needed for good health
Calcium (Ca+)   Potassium (K+)   Magnesium (Mg+)   Zinc (Z+)

Early man ate more than 50% alkaline-forming foods
Modern man eats less than 15% alkaline-forming foods

ing wheat, corn, breads, pastas, and baked goods), refined sugars, and fat. Other acid-forming foods include artificial sweeteners, most processed foods, and dark-colored beans. Although citrus fruits, such as oranges and lemons, contain organic acids and may have an acidic taste, they are not acid forming when metabolized and, in fact, leave an alkaline residue.

HOW DOES INCREASED WHEAT AND SUGAR CONSUMPTION AFFECT pH LEVELS?

Not surprisingly, today's diet, high in wheat, sugar, meat, and oil, but low in fruits and leafy green vegetables, creates imbalance in the form of an acidic pH[11] (and that does not refer to the stomach acidity necessary for digestion, but to overall body fluid acidity in the cells of the blood, tissues, and organs). Acidity in the body is the pathway to inflammation, which, in turn, is the pathway to disease and an unhealthy life. Illness is depressing, further stressing the body and weakening the body, mind, and spirit.

Alkalizing food groups are nutritionally superior to wheat and sugar. Not only do alkaline-forming foods, such as fresh vegetables, fruits, nuts, and seeds, deliver more vitamins, minerals, phytochemicals, and fiber on a per-calorie basis than wheat (refined or whole), but they also provide natural sweetness in the diet without calorie-laden refined sugars. We need to eat more alkalizing foods. For more information, see The Fine Print Appendix E, page 282.

We Eat Too Many Acidic Foods

These are acid-forming (−) food groups that have a pH < 7
Eating too much wheat makes you acidic

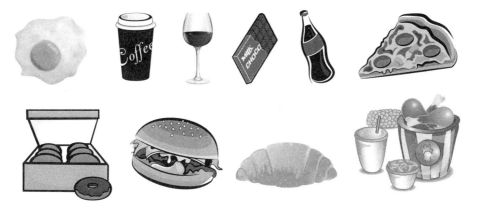

Less than 50% of early man's foods were acid-forming
More than 80% of modern man's foods are acid-forming

HOW DOES AN ACIDIC pH WEAKEN THE IMMUNE SYSTEM?

The body continually strives to balance pH. When body chemistry is not balanced, many problems can occur, much like a swimming pool when the pipes corrode and the surface becomes pitted because the pool's pH has become too acidic or too alkaline. With people, however, the lining of the intestinal tract becomes pitted, allowing bacteria, viruses, yeast, and large food proteins—components that would normally not be allowed to enter—to pass into the blood. These molecules then travel to other tissues and organs, where they are recognized as toxic. In an effort to rid the body of these foreign molecules, white blood cells are released into the blood or affected tissue, creating an inflammatory response.

What causes this inflammatory immune response? Diet, hormones, the physical environment, and stress all trigger inflammation, but diet is the primary trigger. Many experts consider overacidity in the body from the foods we choose to eat to be the principal cause of inflammation. In addition, too much acid will cause the body to excrete alkaline minerals into the blood from the skin, tissue, and joints in an effort to neutralize the acidity. When these alkaline minerals—magnesium, calcium, and potassium—are excreted from the musculoskeletal system, the body's structural integrity weakens, much like the game Jenga, where the building blocks are slowly removed from the tower, piece by piece until the tower eventually collapses.[12] For more information, see The Fine Print Appendix D, page 279.

THE GOOD AND THE BAD OF PROCESSED FOODS

Processed foods are raw food ingredients, such as harvested crops and butchered animal products, which have been transformed into marketable, shelf-stable products ranging from breakfast bars to frozen dinners, snack crackers, canned chicken broth, and processed cheese slices. The advantages of processed foods include ease of distribution (canned broth and tomatoes), convenience (sliced frozen peaches and frozen chopped spinach), consistency (peanut butter and ketchup), and longer shelf life (milk and cookies). The disadvantages of processed foods include lower nutritional value of packaged goods (potato chips), use of additives (high-fructose corn syrup) and preservatives (nitrates), and higher calories per serving than unprocessed foods (apple pie versus an apple).

Acidic pH Weakens Your Immune System

EARLY MAN

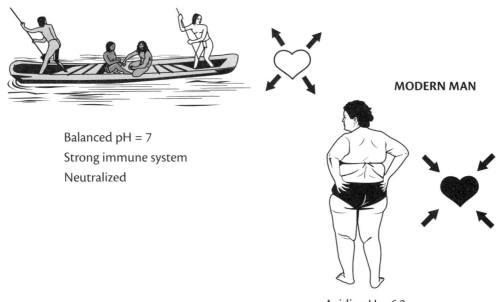

Balanced pH = 7
Strong immune system
Neutralized

MODERN MAN

Acidic pH = 6.2
Weak immune system
Chronic inflammation

Acidic pH robs your bones and organs of these minerals and weakens the body.

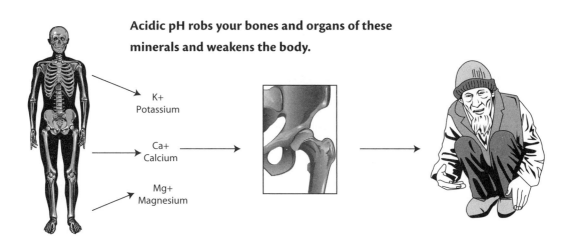

K+
Potassium

Ca+
Calcium

Mg+
Magnesium

HOW DOES INFLAMMATION AFFECT THE IMMUNE SYSTEM?

The human immune system has developed into a collection of 20 trillion highly specialized cells that circulate throughout the body to kill any bad bacteria, virus, yeast, or cancer cells. This highly specialized system can recognize cells as being self (i.e., belonging to the body) and nonself (i.e., a foreign substance). If a cell is recognized as nonself, the immune system begins a series of chemical reactions to destroy the invader cells. Inflammation is the crucial first step in fighting off infection, healing wounds, and maintaining health.

When the immune system is suppressed by such things as diet and stress, there is too little inflammation to fight contagious viruses, bacteria, and parasites, and we contract infectious diseases, such as the flu and pneumonia. When the immune system is overstimulated by such things as diet, prescription medicine, and toxins, there is too much inflammation, and the delicate balance among all of the major systems—endocrine, central nervous, digestive, and cardiovascular/respiratory—is disrupted by this chronic inflammation. In a healthy body, these systems communicate with and respond to one another. With chronic inflammation, this cross-talk no longer works and we develop chronic diseases, such as arthritis, diabetes, cancer, multiple sclerosis, and celiac disease. Therefore, it is important to keep the body neutralized: balanced, strong, and healthy. For more information, see The Fine Print Appendix D, page 279.

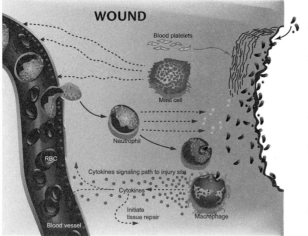

1. Bacteria, viruses, and other toxins enter the body through ingestion or by surface wounds.

2. Blood cells release proteins to clot blood at wound sites.

3. White blood T-cells release messages to the immune system B-cells to produce antibodies to fight the foreign substances (or antigens).

4. Neutrophils secrete substances to destroy and expel antigens.

5. Macrophages secrete hormones called cytokines that signal immune system cells to repair tissue damage through the process of inflammation.

6. This inflammatory response continues until the foreign substances are eliminated and the affected area is repaired.

The Immune System

Over time, those with the strongest immune systems were the only ones to survive, and the immune system eventually developed into 20,000,000,000,000 highly specialized cells.

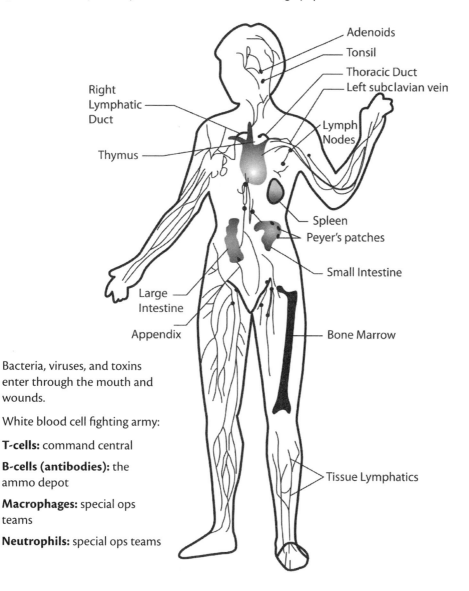

Bacteria, viruses, and toxins enter through the mouth and wounds.

White blood cell fighting army:

T-cells: command central

B-cells (antibodies): the ammo depot

Macrophages: special ops teams

Neutrophils: special ops teams

The organs of the immune system (listed above) either make these highly specialized cells or act as sites for the cells to function

HOW DOES THE FOOD WE EAT OVERSTIMULATE THE IMMUNE SYSTEM?

The gastrointestinal tract is a long muscular tube that starts at the mouth and ends at the anus. Stretched out to its full length, it measures 30 feet long and has a surface area approximately the size of a tennis court (120 × 60 feet). The major function of the gastrointestinal tract is to take in food (ingestion), digest it to extract energy and nutrients (digestion), and expel the remaining waste (defecation).

A very important function of a healthy digestive system is to allow only nutrients (usually in the form of small molecules) to pass from the intestinal wall into the bloodstream. However, when we eat foods to which we are allergic or sensitive, the immune system responds, and an inflammatory reaction occurs when our body defends itself against what it perceives as an invasion. Toxic chemical compounds from the body's white blood cells are released into the blood or affected tissues in an attempt to rid the body of the foreign invaders. In the gastrointestinal tract, this release of chemicals causes inflammation of the gut lining, and as the gut lining becomes inflamed it becomes more difficult to keep large, foreign particles out. Spaces between epithelial and mucosa cells open up, damaging the intestinal wall. When the wall is damaged, larger molecules, such as proteins, bacteria, yeast, and toxins, slip through. The body recognizes these substances as foreign and forms additional antibodies to them in an attempt to expel these intruders from the body, causing more inflammation, further increasing the permeability of the intestinal wall, and resulting in a leaky gut. For more information, see The Fine Print Appendix D, page 279.

The Gastrointestinal Tract

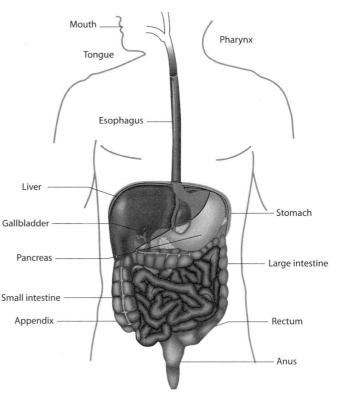

Mouth

Pharynx

Tongue

Esophagus

Liver

Gallbladder

Pancreas

Small intestine

Appendix

Stomach

Large intestine

Rectum

Anus

The Overstimulated Immune System

50% of the immune system surrounds the gastrointestinal tract.

Therefore, what we eat and digest directly affects us!

What do we eat the most of?

Wheat!

The major cause of inflammation in the body is **gluten**, a protein found in **wheat**.

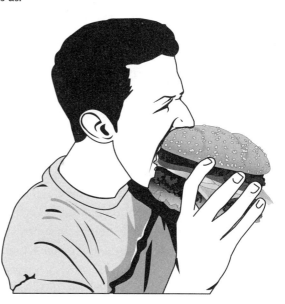

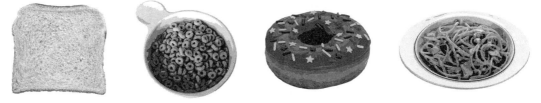

Other Factors Affecting The Immune System

Physical activity	Exercise
Environmental toxins	Pollution, pesticides, chemicals
Stress	Genetics

HOW DOES GLUTEN CAUSE INFLAMMATION?

Leaky gut syndrome is a condition in which the intestinal lining of the digestive tract becomes more permeable, or leakier than normal, due to repeated irritation. The small intestine is designed to allow tiny particles of digested nutrients to pass through its wall and into the bloodstream. These are then distributed for use throughout the body. However, constant irritation can cause the intestinal wall to become more permeable and allow larger, less digested particles and toxins to pass through—thus causing leaky gut syndrome. The body then recognizes these particles as foreign invaders, and the immune system attempts to fight them off. This causes even more inflammation, which sets the stage for various chronic and autoimmune disorders. *The major cause of inflammation and leaky gut syndrome in the body is gluten!*

The term "gluten" refers to the entire protein component of wheat; gliadin is the alcohol-soluble part of gluten that contains toxic components. Our hunter–gatherer ancestors never ate wheat; as a result, the human GI tract, unlike those of cows and sheep, never evolved to digest it. Therefore, undigested molecules of gliadin are resistant to degradation by gastric, pancreatic, and intestinal membrane enzymes, and thus, the gliadin remain in the intestine after gluten ingestion. These peptides (small amino acid chains) are recognized as invaders. Antibodies are released to rid the body of the peptides, and the gut lining becomes inflamed, increasing the permeability of the intestinal wall.[9]

Other contributing factors to gut permeability include: food allergies and sensitivities; stress; heavy alcohol consumption; and the overuse of antibiotics and nonsteroidal anti-inflammatory drugs (NSAIDs), such as aspirin, ibuprofen, and prescription NSAIDs. For more information, see The Fine Print Appendix B, page 270.

Gluten Causes Inflammation

Gliadin peptides remain in the gut and cause the epithelial layer to become more porous, causing increased intestinal permeability

Intestinal Gut

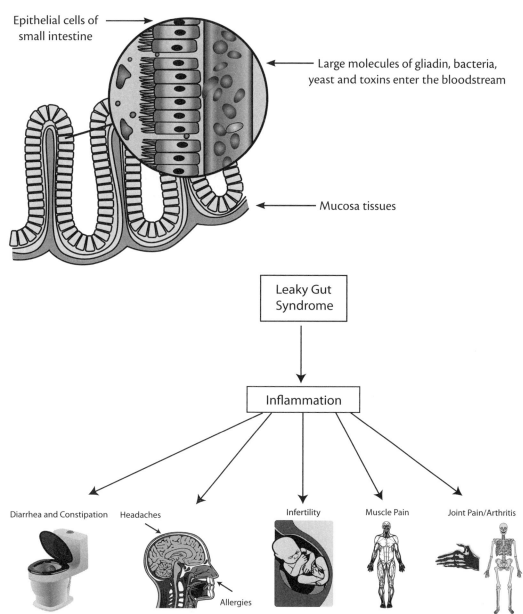

Epithelial cells of small intestine

Large molecules of gliadin, bacteria, yeast and toxins enter the bloodstream

Mucosa tissues

Leaky Gut Syndrome

Inflammation

Diarrhea and Constipation   Headaches   Infertility   Muscle Pain   Joint Pain/Arthritis

Allergies

DOES GLUTEN MAKE EVERYONE'S GUT MORE PERMEABLE?

The human body's strong defensive system creates an inflammatory reaction when gliadin peptides infiltrate the mucosa tissues. T-cells are activated, and the body's innate and adaptive immune system responds. *Wheat makes everyone's gut more permeable because humans cannot adequately break down the gliadin molecules in wheat.*[14] Everyone responds differently to the presence of large proteins in the body, depending on his or her particular genetic profile, stress level, amount of intestinal bacteria, and exposure to toxins. But once these proteins enter the bloodstream and travel to other organs in the body, even healthy, active people can experience diarrhea, headaches, chronic fatigue,[15] arthritis, skin rashes, and allergies.[16] This reaction is called gluten sensitivity.

Gluten sensitivity can be measured in the blood by the presence of elevated gliadin antibody levels.[17] Many gastrointestinal disorders, such as chronic constipation, irritable bowel syndrome, Crohn's disease, and ulcerative colitis, are related to the presence of gliadin antibodies.[18]

One subset of gluten sensitivity is celiac disease, a genetically inherited condition that leads to a reduction in size and flattening in appearance of the villi of the intestinal mucosa. Healthy villi are important because they have several important functions: they release enzymes to digest food, absorb nutrients, and act as a barrier to block toxins from entering the body. Without healthy villi, gastrointestinal distress and, eventually, malnutrition occur, eventually leading to many other serious health complications. There are also some individuals who experience distress when eating gluten but do not suffer damage to the intestinal lining; this sensitivity is referred to as gluten intolerance instead of celiac disease.

Cross Section of the Intestinal Villi

The main functions of the intestinal villi are to

1. Release enzymes to digest food

2. Absorb nutrients

3. Act as a barrier to block toxins from entering the body

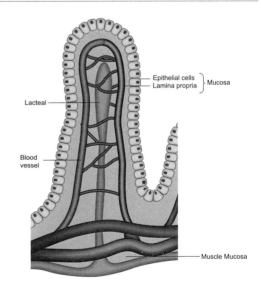

Epithelial cells
Lamina propria } Mucosa

Lacteal

Blood vessel

Muscle Mucosa

GLUTEN SENSITIVITY

Gluten sensitivity has more than 200 symptoms, with the most common being: diarrhea, gas, bloating, vomiting, constipation, nausea, skin irritation, malabsorption, weight loss, anemia, chronic fatigue, weakness, joint pain, muscle cramps, tooth enamel discoloration, thyroid problems, and neurological complaints (including seizures, numbness, migraine headaches, depression, and concentration and memory problems).

The Gluten Sensitivity Spectrum

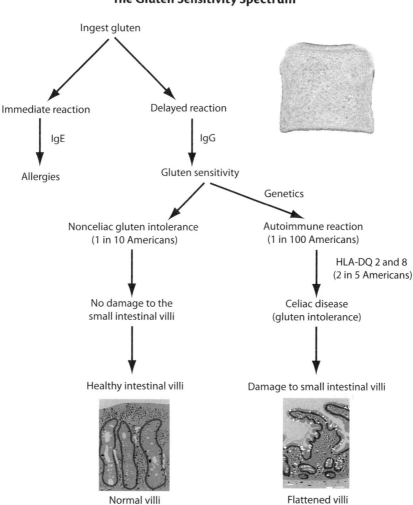

Ingest gluten

Immediate reaction

IgE

Allergies

Delayed reaction

IgG

Gluten sensitivity

Genetics

Nonceliac gluten intolerance
(1 in 10 Americans)

Autoimmune reaction
(1 in 100 Americans)

HLA-DQ 2 and 8
(2 in 5 Americans)

No damage to the
small intestinal villi

Celiac disease
(gluten intolerance)

Healthy intestinal villi

Damage to small intestinal villi

Normal villi

Flattened villi

For more information, see The Fine Print Appendix B, page 270.

HOW CAN YOU EAT SMART?

How can you make the change from a diet comprised of primarily acid-forming foods—wheat, sugar, and animal-based protein—to one that defends your immune system? Luckily, it's simple to change your diet, and you can do it quickly. To be balanced, strong, and healthy, you need to eat more alkaline-forming foods, such as vegetables, fruits, nuts, and seeds, just like your ancestors. The only way to achieve this balance is to know how the foods you eat affect your body's natural chemistry and then choose to eat *more* of those foods that keep you neutralized. You can use pH to measure this effect. Think of your pH as a snapshot of your body's natural chemistry. Wheat, sugar, and processed foods are acidic forming and cause your pH to be acidic. Therefore, it is important to learn to plan and cook meals from whole foods, *not whole wheat*. Whole foods, such as vegetables, fruits, beans, nuts, wild fish, and lean meats, are foods in their original form that help keep your pH balanced.

What does the Gluten-Free Good Health Diet look like? (+) plus (−) = 0. For every meal, divide your plate in half. Fill the left side with alkaline (+) forming foods, which include most vegetables, fruits, and seeds, and many beans and nuts. Fill the right side with acid (−) forming foods, such as wild-caught fish, lean meats, cheese, and whole grains, such as brown rice. By weight, most of your meals will be more acidic, so try to drink at least two cups of green tea each day, as the tea has an alkalizing effect. You should also make sure most of your snacks are alkalizing. If you plan to eat a sugary dessert, balance your day by drinking 8 ounces of lemon water—simply a glass of water with the juice of half a lemon (even though citrus fruits taste acidic, after they're digested they have an alkalizing effect). At the end of every day, your intake of alkalizing and acidic foods should equal 0.

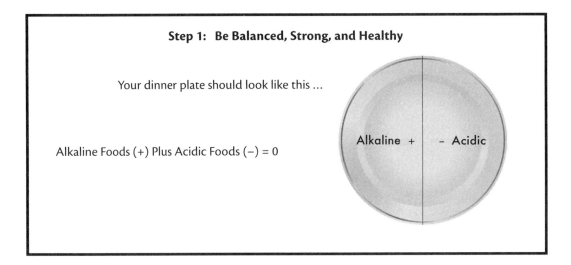

Step 1: Be Balanced, Strong, and Healthy

Your dinner plate should look like this ...

Alkaline Foods (+) Plus Acidic Foods (−) = 0

Alkaline +   − Acidic

Why is it smart to eliminate gluten from your diet? Gluten is a protein found in wheat, rye, barley, and most processed foods. It is not only the number one cause of over acidity in the body (because we eat so much of it daily), but the major cause of inflammation: our body cannot completely break down the gluten protein into digestible molecules. These undigested molecules trigger an inflammatory response in our gut contributing to leaky gut syndrome. Take a minute to realize how much gluten we consume, knowingly and unknowingly, on a daily basis. Common foods that contain gluten include: all wheat (including semolina and spelt), rye and barley breads, pastries, crackers cereals and crumbs; battered and breaded foods; snack mixes and pretzels; prepared frozen entrees; dry soup mixes, prepared broth and bouillons; gravies, sauces, icings and salad dressings that have been thickened; soy sauce; beer (barley); baking ingredients like almond paste, butterscotch morsels and some candies; ice creams; flavored coffees; spice blends; and medications.

By eliminating gluten from your diet, you will not only reduce both acidity and inflammation in your body, but also strengthen the immune system and experience better health. In addition, if you replace wheat-based foods with fruits, vegetables, nuts, and seeds you will lose weight because alkaline-forming foods have fewer calories by weight than foods containing wheat. For more information, see The Fine Print Appendix C, page 277.

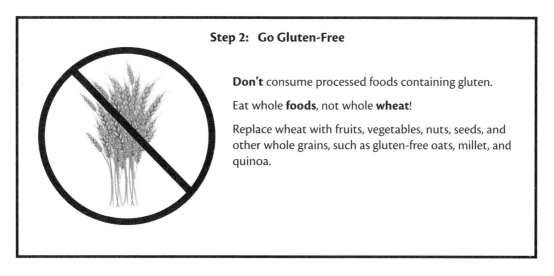

Step 2: Go Gluten-Free

Don't consume processed foods containing gluten.

Eat whole **foods**, not whole **wheat**!

Replace wheat with fruits, vegetables, nuts, seeds, and other whole grains, such as gluten-free oats, millet, and quinoa.

Why does an excess of refined sugars and artificial sweeteners make you inflamed and fat? Sweets should be a treat, not the basis for a meal. Sugar is acidic and it provides no bang for its buck—if a food is loaded with sugar, it's loaded with empty calories. Sugar and artificial sweeteners also disrupt hormone levels, causing the body to store fat—and that makes you fat.

Glucose is the simple sugar your body uses as its primary source of energy. Insulin is the hormone that acts as glucose's gatekeeper, controlling the movement of glucose in and out of cells. It's then either converted to energy or stored in limited quantities, as glycogen in the liver or for future energy needs in the muscles. Once the glycogen levels are filled, any excess glucose is converted to fat and stored in your body's fatty tissue. In a nutshell, sugar, a simple carbohydrate, is fat free, but excess carbohydrates end up as excess fat.

And that's not the worst of it. Any meal or snack that's high in simple carbohydrates, such as pasta, bread, pastries, sweets, cereal, soda, or beer, will generate a rapid rise in your bloodstream's glucose levels. To adjust for this rapid rise, the pancreas secretes insulin into the bloodstream to lower the levels of glucose. Insulin is a storage hormone that is designed to store excess carbohydrate calories in the form of fat. Therefore, the insulin that's stimulated by excess carbohydrate intake aggressively promotes the accumulation of body fat. In other words, when you eat 500 calories of sugar—way more than you need in a day (see page 19)— you're essentially sending your body a hormonal message, via insulin, to store fat.

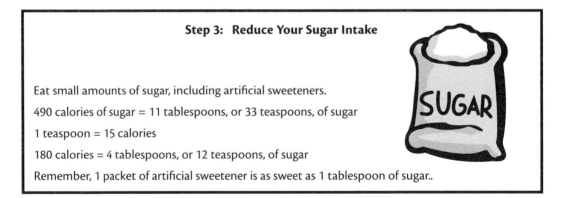

Step 3: Reduce Your Sugar Intake

Eat small amounts of sugar, including artificial sweeteners.

490 calories of sugar = 11 tablespoons, or 33 teaspoons, of sugar

1 teaspoon = 15 calories

180 calories = 4 tablespoons, or 12 teaspoons, of sugar

Remember, 1 packet of artificial sweetener is as sweet as 1 tablespoon of sugar..

What about artificial sweeteners? Artificial sweeteners trick the brain into thinking that sugar is coming. The body gears up for its arrival—and then it doesn't happen. This action affects your hormone levels, which causes the body to burn calories inefficiently, thereby storing excess energy as fat. They also cause excess acidity in the body. Therefore, you should limit your daily intake of artificial sweeteners. If you need to eat something sweet every day, buy good-quality chocolates and eat no more than 1 ounce, or make homemade sweets and limit the portion size to 100 to 150 calories.

WHY SHOULD YOU CHOOSE
THE GLUTEN-FREE GOOD HEALTH DIET?

The *Gluten-Free Good Health Cookbook* **is filled with delicious recipes.** These recipes will inspire you to nourish your body with whole foods that provide balance and satisfaction. In the final recipe chapter, we even offer dessert suggestions that you can enjoy for a weekly treat.

The Gluten-Free Good Health Diet requires thought, planning, and shopping. It's important to stock your house with alkalizing foods and snacks so healthy eating is easy and effortless. Knowing how to cook efficiently is also critical, so your meals can be prepared in the same amount of time it would take you to go out to eat, pick up take-out, or have food delivered. It might seem a lot of time, but all the food planning and preparation will take far less time than the hours you'd otherwise spend in doctors' offices and at the pharmacy, or wasted in bed feeling sick. The Gluten-Free Good Health Diet is all about disease prevention.

The Gluten-Free Good Health Diet is a family activity. Since prehistoric times and the discovery of fire, groups of people have shared food. In those days, mealtimes were events when the whole tribe or community would come together. These group meals not only provided nourishment for survival, but they also strengthened each member's sense of belonging to the group. Instead of watching TV, prepare and serve a family meal together. It's a time for interaction, conversation, sharing, and laughter. The children of families who eat five or more meals together (including breakfast) each week eat more nutritious foods, do better in school, have fewer behavioral problems, are less likely to use drugs and alcohol as teenagers, and are happier than children who usually eat alone.[19]

The Gluten-Free Good Health Diet helps you lose weight. Adherence to any diet is the most important determinant of weight loss. When you eat smart, your food has value. Whole, fresh foods are full of color and flavor. Our recipes are delicious and satisfying. You'll turn your back on mindless eating, like consuming an entire bag of cookies or a microwaved frozen dinner in front of the TV. We encourage you to engage in purposeful planning, shopping, cooking, meal sharing, and eating. You'll naturally eat fewer calories because whole foods contain more water and soluble fiber—both of which are devoid of calories—than processed foods, so you'll feel fuller even though you've consumed fewer calories. Isn't it better to savor the flavor of one delectable melt-in-your-mouth slice of homemade cheesecake than to down a box of store-bought brownies that lack fulfillment? Less is more!

The Gluten-Free Good Health Diet helps you maintain your weight because it isn't just a diet—it's a way of life. Gluten-Free Good Health is a lifestyle, not a fad. It doesn't focus on calorie reduction, carbohydrate restriction, fiber content, or glycemic loads. It isn't centered on one isolated vitamin, mineral, or magical herb that will change your body. The Gluten-

Free Good Health Diet understands that humans evolved to eat whole foods, so whole foods are best for our bodies.

The Gluten-Free Good Health Diet helps you be more successful. Good eating habits and good nutrition are key factors for success. When you feel good, you're better able to make good things happen. A healthy immune system can help you achieve intellectually, professionally, academically, athletically, and socially—at home, work, school, sports, or play. When you feel balanced and strong, you have self-confidence. Who *wouldn't* want to feel good about themselves, their loved ones, their children, and their friends?

The Gluten-Free Good Health Diet is easy to understand. Unlike other diets that are based on gimmicks and hope, this cookbook was developed with an understanding of basic science, proven medical research, and a true love of food and eating—think of it as the PhD meets Julia Child.

Let us show you the gluten-free way to eat smart, strengthen your immune system, and neutralize inflammation.

THE LAST WORD

As you look through the recipe chapters that follow, you'll probably notice that the *Gluten-Free Good Health Cookbook* has a rich variety of both acid- and alkaline-based recipes. We eat and enjoy foods from both groups, and we think you should, too. This is not a diet with a beginning and an end—no 3-week purge with nothing but cucumber juice shakes and cabbage soup; no 30 pages of dull meal plan menus to religiously follow, and no contrived and bizarre recipes (Tofu Sardine Fritters, anyone?) to cook.

The Gluten-Free Good Health Diet doesn't focus on just fat or just calories. It's a marriage between nutrition and deliciously prepared whole foods that help you build a strong immune system and balanced health. We use pH as a scientific tool to measure the success of this marriage, not as a basis for every recipe.

Instead, we want you to enjoy a variety of real, fresh, whole foods, like leafy greens, avocados, oranges, almonds, and wild salmon, and shun heavily processed gimmicks that are so common in other diets, such as dehydrated food shakes and expensive vitamin and mineral supplements. The foundation for all the recipes in this book is whole food. Some of the recipes do add a touch of cream or cheese, but these natural ingredients add flavor and texture and will help make your food delicious and satisfying.

Our strategy for eating is simple, easy to follow, and—most importantly—sustainable. You'll begin to think about the kind of foods you put on your plate, and how much of it you're eating, in order to maintain a neutral pH in your body. Sure, you can eat a reasonable portion of homemade chili or gluten-free pasta, as long as you balance it with lots of vegetables. And you can also enjoy a little dessert every once in a while, but not after every meal. Just be sure to balance that sweet treat with something neutralizing either before or after. You'll feel healthier and you'll find it easier to control your weight.

Of course, we also encourage you to reduce or eliminate gluten from your diet because our research, which you can read more about by looking up the references at the end of this chapter and the book's Fine Print (appendixes), has shown that gluten contributes to inflammation in the body, and that inflammation leads to illness and disease.

CHAPTER 1 REFERENCES

1. Centers for Disease Control and Prevention. 2009. "Chronic Diseases: The Power to Prevent, the Call to Control." http://www.cdc.gov/print.do?url=http://www.cdc.gov/nccdphp/publications/AAG/chronic.htm. Accessed August 13, 2009.

2. Centers for Disease Control and Prevention. 2009. "Fast Stats A to Z." http://www.cdc.gov/nchs/fastats/. Accessed August 13, 2009.

3. Fairweather, D., and Rose, N. 2004. "Women and Autoimmune Disorders." *Emerging Infectious Diseases* 10(11):2005.

4. Campbell, E., J. Weissman, S. Ehringhaus, S. Rao, B. Moy, S. Feibelmann, and S. Goold. 2007. "Institutional Academic-Industry Relationships." *Journal of the American Medical Association* 298:1779–86.

5. Wadley, G., and A. Martin. 2000. "The Origins of Agriculture—A Biological Perspective and a New Hypothesis." *Journal of the Australasian College of Nutritional Health and Environmental Medicine* 19(1):3–12.

6. Eaton, S., and M. Kroner. (1997). "Paleolithic Nutrition Revisited: A Twelve Year Perspective on Its Nature and Implications." *European Journal of Clinical Nutrition* 51:207–216.

7. Putnam, J., J. Allshouse, and L. Kantor. 2002. "U.S. Per Capita Food Supply Trends: More Calories, Refined Carbohydrates, and Fats." *Economic Research Service Food Review* 25(3): 2–15.

8. Rubio-Tapia, A., and J. Murray. 2009. "Increased Prevalence and Mortality in Undiagnosed Celiac Disease." *Gastroenterology* 137(1): 373–374.

9. Tanskanen, Antti, et al. 2001. "Fish Consumption, Depression, and Suicidality in a General Population." *Archives of General Psychiatry* 58(5): 512–13.

10. Myers, G., and P. Davidson. 1998. "Maternal Fish Consumption Benefits Children's Development." *The Lancet* 369, 9561: 537–538.

11. Frassetto L., R. Morris, D. Sellmeyer, and A. Sebastian. 2008. "Adverse Effects of Sodium Chloride on Bone in the Aging Human Population Resulting from Habitual Consumption of Typical American Diets." *Journal of Nutrition*, 138:419–22.

12. Bobkov, V. 1999. "Changes in the Acid-Base Status of the Synovial Fluid in Rheumatoid Arthritis Patients." *Terapevticheski Arkhiv* (Russia).

13. Green, P., and C. Cellier. 2007. "Medical Progress: Celiac Disease." *New England Journal of Medicine* 357:1731–43.

14. Bernardo, D., J.A. Garrote, L. Fernández-Salazar, S. Riestra, E. Arranz. 2007. "Is Gliadin Really Safe for Non-Coeliac Individuals? Production of Interleukin 15 in Biopsy Culture from Non-Coeliac Individuals Challenged with Gliadin Peptides." *Gut* 56(10): 889–890.

15. Amason, J., H. Gudjonsson, J. Freysdottir, I. Jonsdottir, H. Valdimarsson. 1992. "Do Adults with High Gliadin Antibody Concentrations Have Subclinical Gluten Intolerance?" *Gut* 33(2): 194–197.

16. Troncone, R., and Ferguson, A. 1991. "Anti-Gliadin Antibodies." *Journal of Pediatric Gastroenterology and Nutrition* 12:150–158.

17. Wangen, S. 2009. *Healthier Without Wheat*. Seattle, WA: Innate Health Publishing.

18. Koninckx, C., Giliams, J., Polanco, I., Pena, A. 1984. "IGa Antigliadin Antibodies in Celiac and Inflammatory Bowel Disease." *Journal of Pediatric Gastroenterolgy and Nutrition* 3(5):676–682.

19. Eisenberg, M., R. Olson, D. Neumark-Sztainer, M. Story, and L. Bearinger. 2004. "Correlations between Family Meals and Psychosocial Well-Being among Adolescents." *Archives of Pediatric and Adolescent Medicine* 158:792–96.

The Gluten-Free Good Health Diet

CHAPTER 1 EXPLAINED THE IMPORTANT ROLE diet plays in health. If you eat a diet composed primarily of wheat, sugar, and highly processed foods, you'll negatively affect your body's chemistry, resulting in inflammation. Inflammation weakens the immune system. A weak immune system leaves you susceptible to chronic disease. To prevent disease and defend your immune system, you should eat a diet of healthy whole foods, including vegetables, fruits, nuts, seeds, wild fish and lean meat—and not whole wheat. You can use pH to measure the health of your immune system. This chapter will explain how to achieve a healthy acid–alkaline pH balance in your body.

WHAT IS THE GLUTEN-FREE GOOD HEALTH DIET?

The key to defending your immune system is to balance acidic-forming foods with alkalizing-forming foods daily in order to neutralize inflammation in your body. Healthy acidic foods should *not* be avoided, because it's important to eat acidic foods that provide nutrients your body needs, such as lean animal protein, fish, walnuts, black beans, cheese, and brown rice.

Just as importantly, unhealthy acidic foods that comprise almost half of most Americans' daily calories—such as wheat (gluten) and refined sugars (including high-fructose corn syrup)—should be significantly reduced. Of course, people who are gluten intolerant should eliminate wheat altogether. These foods are not only nutrient deficient in relation to their caloric content, but they also contribute to the inflammation, obesity, and chronic illness that affect so many people in this country.[1] If you replace wheat and refined sugar with healthier, less acidic foods, such as seeds, vegetables, fruits, wild fish, and green tea, you'll consume fewer calories per day without going on a diet, you'll feel more energetic and alert, and you'll be happier because you feel good both physically and emotionally.

As noted in Chapter 1, the easiest way to explain the Gluten-Free Good Health Diet is to visualize a serving plate. The foods on the left half of the plate should be alkaline-forming, and the right side of the plate should be filled with acidic-forming foods. The result—a neutralized meal. We've categorized foods in the following manner:

+3 = **Most alkalizing** (lemons, watermelon, leafy green vegetables, pumpkin seeds, olive oil, and miso)

+2 = **Highly alkalizing** (strawberries, grapes, lettuce, sweet potatoes, lentils, almonds, and green tea)

+1 = **Slightly alkalizing** (bananas, oranges, carrots, green peas, tofu, white beans, cashews, and oats)

0 = **Neutral** (dairy)

−1 = **Slightly acidic** (cranberries, corn, red beans, vegetable oil, brown rice, fish, and black tea)

−2 = **Highly acidic** (refined sugar, corn tortilla, peanuts, chicken, coffee, wine, and salad dressings)

−3 = **Most acidic** (artificial sweeteners, fried foods, hydrogenated oils, beef, baked goods, and soda)

See the complete list of alkalizing and acid-forming foods at the end of this chapter.

Ideally, every day's pH intake should equal 0. Remember, liquids count, so if you drink soda, coffee, or wine, you'll need to increase the number of alkalizing-forming foods on the left side of your plate.

An example of a good breakfast option would be oatmeal (1) with a banana (1) and a cup of coffee (−2) at breakfast. By midmorning, you could have a snack of dried apricots and almonds (2) with a cup of green tea (2). Lunch could be a bowl of bean and vegetable soup (0) with gluten-free bread (−3), a few pieces of cheese (−1), and mineral water (0). In the afternoon, another cup of green tea (2), a fresh pear (2), and a little chocolate (−3) would maintain a near-neutral rating and curb your afternoon hunger. For dinner, you might choose roasted wild salmon (−1), sautéed spinach (3) with roasted sweet potatoes (2), a glass of wine (−2), and a serving of store-bought sorbet (−3). At the end of the day, you'd have a neutral rating of 0 and a total of about 2,000 gluten-free calories. To reduce your caloric intake to 1,500, you could eliminate the wine and the sorbet.

We realize that some days will end with a negative rating. Is all lost? No! Just balance your body with either a glass of lemon water or a cup of watermelon. That will get you back on track. Chapter 3 offers a week's worth of immune-strengthening menus, and remember, all the recipes in this book are gluten free.

We recommend eliminating all soda—both diet and regular—from your diet and replacing it with water, sparkling water, and herbal and green teas. A regular soda has the equivalent of 9 teaspoons of sugar, and a diet soda has the equivalent of 6 packets of Equal. Just imagine allowing yourself or your children to put 9 teaspoons of sugar or 6 packets of

NEUTRALIZING MEAL SUGGESTIONS

Pre-Breakfast

Drink 8 ounces of room-temperature water with the juice of half a fresh lemon (+). In order to maximize the cleansing, neutralizing, and stimulating benefits lemon water has on the digestive system, it's important to drink lemon water first thing in the morning—when your stomach is empty—so it doesn't mix with any other food or liquid.

Breakfast Ideas

A tropical fruit smoothie made with orange juice and unsweetened yogurt or soy milk (+) and coffee (–)

Sesame oatmeal rolls with an egg, one piece of bacon (–), a banana (+), lemon water (+), and black tea (–)

Oatmeal (+), raisins (+), a fresh orange (+), and coffee (–)

Buckwheat pancakes (+), sautéed pears (+), maple syrup (–), and black tea (–)

Morning and Afternoon Snack

Green tea (+), a handful of sunflower seeds (+), and an apple (+)

Lemon water (+), a small sweet treat (a cookie or some chocolate) (–), and a handful of almonds (+)

Watermelon (+)

Hummus (+) with rice crackers (–) and cut vegetables (+)

Lunch and Dinner

A fresh green salad (+) with wild salmon (–) or roast chicken (–)

Vegetable bean soup (+) with rice crackers (–) and cheese (–)

Roast chicken (–), a sweet potato (+), and asparagus (+)

Beef (–) and broccoli (+) stir fry with brown rice (–)

Barbecued pork (–), pinto beans (–), and grilled vegetables (+)

Spinach (+) and goat cheese (–) pie

Lunch Ideas for Kids

Chicken enchiladas (–) with salsa (+) and tossed salad (+)

A nut butter sandwich on gluten-free bread (–) and fresh fruit (+)

A chicken Caesar salad (0) with fresh fruit (+) and a gluten-free cookie (–)

Baked ham (–), a baked potato (+), peas (+), and a 100 percent frozen-fruit popsicle (+)

Yogurt (–) with fresh fruit (+) and a gluten-free pumpkin muffin (–)

Grilled cheese on gluten-free bread (–), carrot and celery sticks (+), and baked chips (+)

WHY ARE ACIDIC LEMONS ALKALINE-PRODUCING?

The answer is simple, actually: When you digest a lemon or lemon juice, it produces alkaline residue. That's why lemons are classified as an alkaline food. When you digest foods, they are chemically oxidized ("burned") to form water, carbon dioxide, and an inorganic compound. The alkaline or acidic nature of the inorganic compound formed determines whether the food is alkaline or acid-producing. If it contains more sodium, potassium, or calcium, it's classified as an alkaline food. If it contains more sulphur, phosphate, or chloride, it's classified as an acidic food.

Sweet'N Low in a glass of iced tea. You'd scream, "Stop!" So stop. Sweeteners, whether they are real or artificial, affect your hormones and cause your body to store energy as fat. In addition, soda contains phosphoric acid, which is extremely acid-forming.

You should also be cautious about sports and energy drinks. They are acid-forming. Most have similar sugar levels as soda, if not higher, and many contain caffeine, which is an addictive drug. Consuming more than 300 milligrams of caffeine daily can cause the body to lose calcium; this can lead to bone loss over time.[2] Sparkling water and green tea are much healthier alternatives. Even black iced teas are better choices—if they are unsweetened or if only small amounts of sweeteners are added.

GETTING STARTED

The Gluten-Free Good Health Diet emphasizes fresh, whole foods, so our recipes use few processed foods. The processed foods we do use are usually foods that have been minimally processed to lengthen their shelf life and make transportation easier. Examples are frozen plain vegetables and fruits, rice, broth, canned tomatoes, canned beans, and corn tortillas. We do not use frozen or shelf-stable prepared entrees, nor do we buy a lot of packaged shelf-stable snacks.

We do buy certain high-quality processed convenience foods, such as gluten-free pasta, organic tomato sauce, nut and rice crackers, yogurt, and frozen sorbets. Reducing the number of items you buy in the supermarket will reduce the amount of time you spend shopping. Currently, the average supermarket store size is 47,000 square feet and contains more than 47,000 items.[3] If you spend most of your time in the store buying whole foods, which are usually found in its perimeter, you'll only need to zip down the grocery and frozen-food aisles to pick up a few specific items, such as whole grains, green tea, and coconut milk. See Chapter 4 for more information to help you get started.

HOW DO YOU DETERMINE PORTION SIZE?

Serving sizes are the food portions recommended by the USDA Pyramid Guide and the serving sizes of food mentioned on the food's Nutrition Facts label. The following are examples of recommended portion sizes:

- 1 piece medium-sized fruit (such as an apple, orange, banana, or pear)
- ¾ cup (6 ounces) of 100 percent fruit or vegetable juice
- ½ cup cut-up fruit
- ½ cup of raw, cooked, or canned frozen fruits or vegetables
- 1 cup of raw, leafy vegetables (such as lettuce and spinach)
- ¼ cup dried fruit or nuts (such as raisins and almonds)
- ½ cup cooked or canned legumes (such as beans and peas)
- 1 slice bread
- ½ cup cooked cereal, like oatmeal
- ½ cup rice or pasta
- 1 cup cold cereal
- 3 ounces meat, poultry, or fish
- 2 tablespoons nut butter (peanut butter)
- 1 cup milk or yogurt
- 1½ ounces hard cheese
- 2 processed cheese slices
- 1 egg
- 1 teaspoon fat or oil
- Alcohol: 5 ounces wine, 12 ounces beer, 1 ounce distilled spirits

To simplify the process of balancing alkaline and acid foods, we present the following visual representations of portion sizes:

VEGETABLES AND FRUIT

One serving looks like . . .

    1 cup salad greens = a baseball

    1 baked potato = a fist

    1 piece of medium-size fruit = a baseball

    ½ cup fresh fruit = ½ baseball

    ¼ cup dry fruit = a large egg

BEANS, NUTS, AND SEEDS

One serving looks like . . .

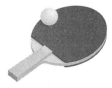

    ½ cup beans = ½ baseball

    ¼ cup nuts = a large egg

    2 tablespoons nut butter = a ping-pong ball

FATS

One serving looks like . . .

    1 teaspoon butter, margarine, spread, or oil = 1 die

GRAIN PRODUCTS

One serving looks like . . .

    1 cup cereal flakes = a fist

    1 pancake = a compact disc

    ½ cup cooked rice, pasta, or potato = ½ baseball

    1 slice bread = a cassette tape

MEAT AND MEAT ALTERNATIVES

One serving looks like . . .

    3 ounces meat, fish, and poultry = a deck of cards

    3 ounces grilled/baked fish = a checkbook

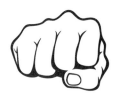

DAIRY AND CHEESE

One serving looks like . . .

    1½ ounces cheese = 4 stacked dice (2 cheese slices)

    ½ cup ice cream = ½ baseball

GETTING YOUR MINERALS

Minerals act as catalysts for many biological reactions within the human body. These reactions are vital for good health; they include: immune defense, nervous system activity, energy production, bone flexibility, and the digestion and use of vitamins in foods. Our bodies cannot manufacture minerals, so it's important to eat a wide variety of plants and protein to ensure you get adequate levels. The following is a list of the most commonly consumed foods for key minerals.

- Calcium: almonds, amaranth, beans, bok choy, dairy products, leafy green vegetables (spinach, kale, Swiss chard, broccoli), salmon, and tofu
- Magnesium: almonds, amaranth, avocados, beans, Brazil nuts, buckwheat, chocolate, miso, oysters, peanuts, pumpkin seeds, quinoa, spinach, and sunflower seeds
- Potassium: apricots, avocados, bananas, beans, beets, bok choy, broccoli, Brussels sprouts, cantaloupe, chocolate, clams, figs, pomegranates, oranges, potatoes, quinoa, tomatoes, water chestnuts, and yogurt
- Zinc: beans, beef, chicken, crab, lamb, lentils, oysters, pumpkin seeds, and turkey[4]

HOW DO YOU USE PORTION SIZE TO (+) PLUS (–) = 0?

If you plan to eat 6 ounces of salmon (2 serving sizes) and ½ cup brown rice (1 serving size) on the right side of your plate, you'll need to balance it with at least 1 cup of cooked broccoli (2 servings) and ½ cup of another vegetable, such as raw carrots, or ½ cup cut-up fresh fruit, such as strawberries (1 serving).

On days when nothing but a grilled medium-rare steak and hearty merlot will do, make sure to grill up plenty of vegetables and potatoes right alongside that steak in order to balance your meal. (See Chapter 7 in this book for great vegetable recipes.) Finish the meal with fresh-cut watermelon and neutralize yourself further with a glass of fresh lemon water.

We have found that breakfasts tend to be more acidic (eggs, bacon, gluten-free toast, gluten-free pancakes, gluten-free granola, sweetened yogurt, coffee, and black tea), so we drink green tea throughout the day and eat nuts and fruits for an alkalizing snack. Lunches are a balance of vegetables, fruits, grains, and protein. Dinners tend to feature more vegetables than fruits, and they'll end up slightly more acidic if we drink wine or eat dessert. We try to neutralize it all with fresh lemon water in the morning, but a little lemon water anytime during the day will work, too. The important thing is to make lemon water a part of your daily routine.

The key to (+) plus (–) = 0 is to try to balance every meal as much as possible. When you're first starting out, it may be easier to think about balancing the entire day instead—it's considerably simpler. For example, if you have a cheese sandwich for lunch and then eat alkalizing snacks, such as cut carrots and celery, sliced fruit, or a handful of almonds, later in the afternoon, you'll still find it pretty easy to reach that balance by the end of the day.

THE GLUTEN-FREE GOOD HEALTH DIET RECOMMENDED CALORIE INTAKE

- **40 percent carbohydrate**: Predominately complex carbohydrates; try to consume locally and/or organically grown carbs; and make sure they're gluten-free. Find carbohydrate calories in vegetables, fruits, and whole grains. Remember: Alcoholic drinks are carbohydrate calories, too, and so are sugars.

- **35 percent protein**: Both animal- and plant-based protein (at first this number may seem high, but most vegetables and many fruits contain protein); be sure to buy protein sources that don't contain antibiotics or hormones; if possible, try to buy organic products; if buying fish, choose wild-caught types; meats should be lean; and beans, tofu, low-fat dairy, and nuts are all great sources of protein.

- **25 percent fats**: Predominately monosaturated or polyunsaturated fats, such as olive oil, canola oil, flax seed oil, avocados, and nut butters.

- **Sugar intake**: Less than 10 percent of total calories, or up to 4 packets of artificial sweeteners.

If you eat 2,000 calories per day, a good breakdown is as follows:

- 800 calories from carbohydrates (no more than 200 calories from sugar)
- 700 calories from protein
- 500 calories from fat

Daily calorie needs are not one-size-fits-all. People who are small, female, older, or less

GREEN TEA

What makes green tea so special? The secret of green tea lies in the fact it is rich in catechin polyphenols—particularly epigallocatechin gallate (EGCG). EGCG is a powerful antioxidant. Not only does it inhibit the growth of cancer cells, but it is also effective in lowering LDL cholesterol levels and inhibiting the abnormal formation of blood clots (thrombosis). The latter takes on added importance when you consider that thrombosis is the leading cause of heart attacks and stroke. Research has also shown that green tea helps boost the immune system, inhibit intestinal inflammation, and lower stress hormone levels.[5] Green tea is delicious both cold and hot, and there are many different types. If you're new to tea, try a honey-lemon green tea or a jasmine green tea. For an earthier flavor, try a Japanese green tea.

OMEGA-3 FATS

Researchers believe that omega-3 fats play an important role in controlling inflammation. But most Americans do not get enough omega-3 fats from their diet. The main reason is the ratio of two different families of polyunsaturated oils in the diet. The two families are called omega-3 and omega-6 fats, and Americans tend to eat far more omega-6 fats than omega-3 fats—by a ratio of 12 to 1!

Some researchers believe that for people with inflammatory conditions, a ratio of 3-to-1 may be beneficial in decreasing inflammation. This is because certain inflammatory substances (prostaglandins) are made out of these fats, and the ones made out of omega-6 fats are much more inflammatory than the ones made out of omega-3 fats.

To increase omega-3 fats in your diet, replace corn oil, which is high in omega-6 and very low in omega-3, when you are cooking and baking with either olive oil (neutral, so it displaces the high omega-6 oils) or canola oil (an oil with a better ratio of omega-3 and omega-6 fat).[7] In addition, it's important to eat foods that are high in omega-3 fats, such as flax seeds, walnuts, salmon, soybeans, cauliflower, and cabbage.

active usually need fewer daily calories than people who are tall, male, younger, or active. To get a better indication of your personal daily calorie needs, try the American Cancer Society's interactive calorie calculator, which you can find on its Web site at http://www.cancer.org/docroot/PED/content/PED_6_1x_Calorie_Calculator.asp. You'll enter your current weight, gender, and activity level into the calculator, and it will recommend the right calorie amount for you if you wish to lose weight or maintain your weight. If you want to lose weight, the calculator gives this simple formula: To lose 1 pound per week, you need to create a deficit of 500 calories per day. You can do this one of two ways: by eating 500 fewer calories, or by eating 250 fewer calories a day (for example, eliminate a 20-ounce bottle of regular soda) and burning an extra 250 calories through physical activity (for example, a 2.5-mile walk).

OTHER NUTRITIONAL AND ACTIVITY RECOMMENDATIONS

A strong immune system is the key to preventing disease. These additional lifestyle guidelines promote good health.

> **Herbal or green tea:** 2–4 cups per day.
>
> **Sodium intake:** Up to 2,400 milligrams per day.
>
> **Alcohol:** A maximum of 1 drink per day for women and 2 drinks per day for men.
>
> **Minimum physical activity:** Daily moderate activity for 30 minutes per day and strength training for a total of 90 minutes per week (two 45-minute sessions of weight-based exercise or yoga).

EXERCISE

Exercise is potent medicine. It releases compounds, such as endorphins, into the blood that naturally reduce inflammation. Exercise helps lower c-reactive proteins (which rise when inflammation occurs), regulate insulin levels, and build muscle, which helps the body regulate weight. "Mindful" exercise combined with deep breathing, such as yoga, walking, tai chi, or Pilates, has the double benefit of reducing psychological stress. Physical activity can help you avoid developing functional limitations and can improve your physical function. And remember—physical activity doesn't have to be strenuous in order to be beneficial.

WHERE TO BEGIN? TEST YOUR pH

You should test your pH levels to determine if your body's pH needs immediate attention. By using pH test strips, you can determine your pH factor quickly and easily in the privacy of your own home. If your urinary pH is between 6.5 and 7.2, your body is functioning within a healthy range (it will be lower in the morning). If your saliva stays between 6.5 and 7.5 all day, your body is functioning within a healthy range. The best time to test your pH is about 1 hour before a meal (first thing in the morning) or 2 hours after a meal (before going to bed). When you first start the Gluten-Free Good Health Diet, you should test your pH daily for 2 weeks.

Where can you buy pH strips? You can purchase pH strips at health food stores, Whole Foods Market stores, Sprouts Farmers Markets, or online at www.amazon.com and www.ph-ion.com

Urine pH: Urine testing indicates how well your body is excreting acids and assimilating minerals, especially calcium, magnesium, sodium, and potassium. These minerals function as buffers. Buffers are substances that help maintain and balance the body against the introduction of too much acidity or too much alkalinity. Even with the proper amounts of buffers, acid or alkaline levels can become extreme. When the body ingests or produces too many of these acids or alkalis, it must excrete the excess. The urine is the perfect way for the body to remove any excess acids or alkaline substances that cannot be buffered. If your average urine pH is below 6.5, you are too acidic and the body's buffering system is overwhelmed. You need to neutralize and eat more alkalizing foods.

Saliva pH: Saliva pH testing indicates the activity of digestive enzymes in the body. These enzymes are primarily manufactured by the stomach, liver, and pancreas. If your saliva pH is too high (> 7.5), you may experience excess gas, constipation, and production of yeast, mold, and fungus. If your saliva pH is too low (< 6.5), your body may be producing too many acids or may be overwhelmed by acids because it has lost the ability to adequately remove them through the urine. Although the saliva also uses buffers just like the urine, it relies on this process to a much lesser degree. Therefore, the pH of saliva offers a window through which you can see the overall pH balance in your body.

What should you do if your pH is below 6.5? Fresh lemon water is extremely alkalizing. If your body is acidic, drink a glass of room-temperature lemon water, preferably in the morning. Squeeze the juice of half a fresh lemon (at room temperature) into 8 ounces of room-temperature, filtered, neutral water (pH = 7). Be sure that you get the juice from fresh lemons, and not bottled, reconstituted juice. (Reconstituted lemon juice is made by adding water back into concentrated lemon juice. Because it's a processed food, reconstituted lemon juice requires the flavor to be adjusted in order to maintain a uniform flavor, and preservatives are added to maintain color and freshness.) Eliminate all soda (diet or regular) and wheat (refined or whole) from your diet, and reduce your daily consumption of refined sugars to 180 calories (12 teaspoons), including baked goods, ketchup, and candy. Next, balance your alkaline-forming and acid-forming foods so (+) plus (–) = 0 on a daily basis.

Once you've balanced your pH, continue to test it once or twice a week—preferably Monday and Friday—in order to maintain that balance. If you find yourself becoming slightly acidic, just follow the basic Gluten-Free Good Health Diet principles listed at the end of the chapter. The beauty of this diet is its sustainability: It is easy to follow, doesn't require any gimmicks, and is filled with satisfying and delicious foods. Once you've been neutralized, you'll want to stay balanced because it will make you feel better, healthier, and stronger.

SPICE IT UP

Spices play an important role in eating smart. Not only do they add variety and flavor to foods, but most herbs and spices are alkaline-forming and help neutralize the foods they are prepared with. Pasta with tomatoes and basil, stir-fried beef with garlic and ginger, roast turkey with thyme and sage, cilantro and chili powder in chicken enchiladas, and cinnamon and nutmeg in apple pie are classic examples of how herbs and spices add not only flavor but also alkalizing benefits to some of our favorite acidic foods.

In addition, many spices act as anti-inflammatory agents, reducing swelling and discomfort. The recipes in this book use these ingredients not only as flavor components, but also as health enhancers. Inflammation is suspected to play a key role in heart disease, cancer, atherosclerosis, arthritis, asthma, allergies, and more. Spicing up your food can help you keep those diseases at bay. The following are some top anti-inflammatory herbs and spices:

Ginger	Cinnamon	Cardamom	Cloves
Turmeric	Rosemary	Chives	Garlic
Black pepper	Basil	Cilantro	Parsley

ALKALINE AND ACID-FORMING FOODS[6,7]

Food Category	Lowest Alkaline +1	Alkaline +2	Most Alkaline +3
Sweeteners	Molasses, raw honey, raw sugar, stevia	Fructose, maple syrup, rice syrup	
Fruits	Apricots, avocado, blueberries, cherries, coconut, nectarines, peaches, pineapple, rhubarb	Apples, bananas, blackberries, dates, figs, grapes, melons, oranges, papaya, pears, raisins, raspberries, strawberries	Grapefruit, kiwi, lemon, lemon juice, lime, lime juice, mango, papaya, tangerine, watermelon
Vegetables	Bean sprouts, Brussels sprouts, cabbage, carrots, cucumbers, green peas, mushrooms, olives, potato, sour pickles, snow peas, tomatoes	Artichokes, beets, carob, cauliflower, eggplant, jicama, lettuce greens, okra, peppers, squash, sweet potato, turnips, watercress, zucchini	Asian vegetables, asparagus, broccoli, celery, collards, daikon, dandelion greens, edible flowers, endive, fennel, kale, garlic, mustard greens, nori, onions, parsnips, parsley, radish, raw spinach, rutabagas, wild greens
Beans and legumes	Mung bean, navy bean, soybean, tempeh, tofu, white bean	Lentils, soy sauce, tamari	Miso
Grains and cereals	Amaranth, buckwheat, millet, oats, quinoa, wild rice		
Nuts and seeds	Cashews, macadamia nuts, sunflower seeds, sesame seeds	Almonds, almond milk, flax seeds, spice seeds	Pumpkin seeds, chestnuts
Fats and oils	Avocado oil, canola oil, coconut oil	Flax seed oil	Olive oil
Eggs and dairy		Breast milk	
Beverages	Apple cider, fresh fruit juices, mineral water	Fresh vegetable juice, green tea	Herbal teas, ginger tea, lemon water
Other foods	Baked potato chips, mustard, tomato sauce	All herbs, pepper, dry spices including chili pepper, cinnamon, coriander, curry	Apple cider vinegar, baking powder, baking soda, green herbs, ginger root, horseradish, sea salt, seaweed

Food Category	Lowest Acid –1	Acid –2	Most Acid –3
Sweeteners	Processed honey	White sugar, brown sugar	Nutrasweet, Equal, aspartame, Sweet 'n Low, Splenda
Fruits	Cranberries, plums, pomegranates, prunes		
Vegetables	Fresh corn		Chocolate, French fries
Beans and legumes	Beans: black, fava, garbanzo, green, kidney, lima, pinto, wax, yellow; soy cheese; soy milk	Baked beans	
Grains and cereals	Brown rice, sorghum, teff	Barley, cornmeal, rye flour, white rice	Cakes, cookies, crackers, pasta, pastries, pies, sweetened cereals, wheat flour
Nuts and seeds	Pine nuts	Pecans, pistachios, peanuts	Soy nuts, hazelnuts, walnuts
Fats and oils	Butter, corn oil, margarine, sesame oil, sunflower oil, vegetable oil	Lard, peanut oil, soybean oil	Cottonseed oil, hydrogenated oils
Meats	Clams, cold water fish, duck, game meat, venison	Buffalo, chicken, lamb, rabbit, turkey	Bacon, beef, cold cuts, pork, shellfish, veal
Eggs and dairy	Butter, buttermilk, cottage cheese, egg whites, goat milk, kefir, ricotta, whey, yogurt	Raw milk, most soft cheeses, whole eggs	Aged cheese, cream, egg yolks, frozen desserts, pasteurized milk, sweetened yogurt
Beverages	Black tea, tap water	Coffee, wine, rice milk	Beer, sweetened juices, hot cocoa, liquor, soft drinks
Other foods	Mayonnaise, most vinegars	Ketchup, popcorn, salad dressings	Aspirin, canned foods, chips, fried foods, iodized table salt, manufactured drugs, pretzels, processed foods, yeast

ALKALINE AND ACID-FORMING FOODS[6,7]

SUMMARIZING THE GLUTEN-FREE GOOD HEALTH DIET PRINCIPLES

1. Test your pH.

2. Eat whole foods.

3. Alkaline foods + acid-forming foods = 0.

4. Go gluten-free.

5. Significantly reduce your intake of sugar and artificial sweeteners.

6. Eliminate diet and regular sodas, and drink more water and green tea.

7. Eat only minimally processed foods, such as frozen plain vegetables and fruits, canned tomatoes, and soup broth.

8. Start each day with fresh lemon water.

9. Learn to cook.

10. Enjoy your food.

CHAPTER 2 REFERENCES

1. Giugliano, D., Ceriello, A., and Esposito, F. 2006. "The Effects of Diet on Inflammation: Emphasis on the Metabolic Syndrome." *Journal of the American College of Cardiology*, 48: 677–85.

2. Rapuri, P., Gallagher, J. Kinyamu, H., Ryschon, K. 2001. "Caffeine Intake Increases the Rate of Bone Loss in Elderly Women and Interacts with Vitamin D Receptor Genotypes." *American Journal of Clinical Nutrition*, 74:694–700.

3. Food Marketing Institute. 2007. Supermarket Facts: Industry Overview 2008. http://www. fmi.org/facts_figs/?fuseaction=superfact. Accessed August 1, 2009.

4. Foods Reference Library, www.wholehealthmd.com.

5. Green Tea. 2007. University of Maryland Medical Center. http://www.umm.edu/altmed/ articles/green-tea-000255.htm. Accessed August 7, 2009.

6. Brown, S. and Triveri, L. 2006. *The Acid Alkaline Food Guide*. Garden City Park, NY: Square One Publishers.

7. Vasey, C. 2005. *The Acid-Alkaline Diet for Optimum Health: Restore Your Health by Creating pH Balance in Your Diet*. Rochester, VT: Healing Arts Press.

CHAPTER 3

Daily Gluten-Free Good Health

CHAPTER 2 INTRODUCED YOU to the 10 Gluten-Free Good Health principles.

1. Test your pH.

2. Eat whole foods.

3. Alkaline foods + acid-forming foods = 0.

4. Go gluten-free.

5. Significantly reduce your intake of sugar and artificial sweeteners.

6. Eliminate diet and regular sodas, and drink more water and green tea.

7. Eat only minimally processed foods, such as frozen plain vegetables and fruits, canned tomatoes, and soup broth.

8. Start each day with fresh lemon water.

9. Learn to cook.

10. Enjoy your food.

Just as it's important to monitor your pH in order to determine the health of your immune system, it is important to learn how to cook whole, fresh, and delicious food so you can actually build and maintain a healthy immune system in the first place. This chapter provides the framework for the Gluten-Free Good Health Diet. It discusses how to think about food on a daily basis, how to plan your eating and your meals, and it offers several simple whole-food recipes you can make every week.

The hardest part of any change is getting started. Following is an example of a seven-day Gluten-Free Good Health menu that can help you start your journey toward a strong, healthy, and balanced life. All the recipes included in the menu can be found in this book. In addition, we recommend you follow the daily Gluten-Free Good Health Diet practices listed at the end of this chapter to ensure your success.

SEVEN DAYS OF EATING SMART

	Breakfast	Lunch	Dinner
Day 1	Fruit smoothie Coffee or tea	Grilled cheese on gluten-free bread with sprouts, tomatoes, and sliced avocado Water or seltzer	White chicken chili with a mixed green salad Water, tea, or wine
Day 2	Fried egg and bacon sandwich on a sesame oatmeal roll with seasonal fresh fruit Coffee or tea	Bean soup with rice crackers and cheese Water or seltzer	Pork tenderloin with southern rub, grilled or roasted vegetables, and brown rice Water, tea, or wine
Day 3	Oatmeal and fresh fruit (such as bananas or berries) Coffee or tea	Grilled chicken with sweet potatoes and seasonal vegetables Water or seltzer	Gluten-free pasta with tomato sauce and bison meatballs with a mixed green salad Water, tea, or wine
Day 4	Scrambled eggs and gluten-free toast with seasonal fresh fruit Coffee or tea	Spinach and goat cheese pie with a gluten-free pumpkin muffin Water or seltzer	Marinated beef steaks with white bean and tomato salad, and ratatouille Water, tea, or wine
Day 5	Granola, yogurt, and fresh fruit (such as bananas or berries) Coffee or tea	Beef fajitas with brown rice, salsa, guacamole, and seasonal vegetables Water or seltzer	Skillet shrimp with fire-roasted tomatoes, quinoa, and steamed vegetables Water, tea, or wine
Day 6	Egg white–cheese omelet on a corn tortilla with salsa and sliced fresh avocado Coffee or tea	Baby greens with balsamic vinaigrette and roasted wild salmon Water or seltzer	Turkey scaloppini with mashed potatoes and roasted vegetables Water, tea, or wine
Day 7	Buckwheat pancakes or waffles and sautéed seasonal fruit (such as apples, pears, and bananas) Coffee or tea	Mediterranean plate with gluten-free crackers and sugar snap peas Water or seltzer	Grilled fish with grilled vegetables and sweet potatoes Water, tea, or wine

REAL-LIFE GLUTEN-FREE GOOD HEALTH

The following testimonials are from our students, readers, and clients. We've changed their names and careers, but their stories are real.

John is a 45-year-old sales executive who has suffered from allergies and nasal congestion for his entire life. Eventually, he consulted doctors about his allergy problems. They conducted extensive blood and skin allergy testing that was inconclusive. After six weeks on the Gluten-Free Good Health Diet, John experienced significantly fewer allergy attacks and an overall feeling of better health. Now a full year after starting the diet, his health is still much better, and he experiences far fewer colds or sicknesses of any type. He easily keeps a gluten-free diet at home, but he finds it more challenging when traveling on business. Fortunately, there's a growing awareness of gluten sensitivity and gluten-free options at more restaurants, so it's becoming easier to find gluten-free options when dining out

Susan is a retiree who has suffered from abdominal pain, bloating, constipation, and weight issues for the past 20 years. After two weeks on the Gluten-Free Good Health Diet, her gastrointestinal pain and constipation were gone. Within two months, Susan lost 10 pounds. Now a year later, Susan has continued to keep the weight off and remains in good health and free of pain.

Maria is a 56-year-old housewife who has experienced acid reflux for many years. After three days on the Gluten-Free Good Health Diet, she noticed a reduction in the amount of reflux and sour stomach she encountered. Within six months, Maria was able to stop taking a prescription acid reducer and now just uses an over-the-counter medication occasionally. She doesn't find it difficult to stay on the diet, and she carefully balances each of her meals and snacks. For example, she adds dark leafy lettuce, sprouts, and avocado to turkey sandwiches made with gluten-free bread, and adds slices of lemon or cucumber to her glasses of water throughout the day.

Lisa is a 38-year-old schoolteacher with a husband and two teenagers. She has had dry, flaky skin rashes for her entire life; often, the rashes appear on her face and arms. Lisa's mother died of stomach cancer in her fifties. After testing negative for celiac disease, Lisa went on a gluten-free diet anyway. Her rashes disappeared immediately. If she happens to "cheat" with a piece of pizza or a slice of birthday cake containing gluten, the rash will return within 24 hours. Now that she knows she's gluten sensitive, she has eradicated gluten from her diet, and she also tries her best to balance her pH at home and school by drinking lots of lemon water and green tea throughout the day, and eating fresh fruits and/or vegetables at every meal.

BREAKFAST

The most important thing about breakfast is to eat a combination of foods: complex carbohydrates for energy, lean protein for physical and mental stability throughout the morning, and some fat so you'll feel full until lunch. Research shows that people who eat breakfast have more nutritious diets, better eating habits, and are less likely to be overweight.[1]

EASY SCRAMBLED EGGS

Serves 2

   3 large eggs

   1 tablespoon nonfat milk, soy milk, water, or olive oil

   1 teaspoon butter, for frying

   Freshly ground sea salt and black pepper

1. Preheat a small, nonstick frying pan over medium-high heat. In a small bowl, whisk together the eggs with the milk for 30 seconds.

2. Melt the butter in the frying pan. As the very last of the butter liquefies, add the egg mixture. Reduce the heat to medium.

3. Do not stir immediately; instead, wait until the first hint of setting begins. Using a spatula or a flat wooden spoon, push the eggs toward the center of the pan while tilting the pan to redistribute any of the remaining liquid.

4. Keep tilting the pan as the eggs continue to set. Break apart any large pieces that form with your spoon or spatula. You will come to a point where the push-to-center technique stops cooking any remaining runny parts of the egg. At that point, flip over all the eggs, and allow them to cook 15 to 25 seconds longer. Transfer the eggs to serving plates. Season with the salt and pepper, to taste.

Variations

- For an egg-white scramble, use 6 egg whites in place of the 3 large eggs.

- To make an omelet: In Step 4, do not continue to stir the eggs; instead, let the eggs settle. When they are moist on top and set on the bottom, carefully fold half the eggs on top of the other half, or roll it over. For an easy, nontraditional omelet, carefully turn the eggs over and cook an additional 30 seconds.

- To make a traditional cheese omelet: When the eggs are moist on top and set on the bottom, sprinkle 2 tablespoons of shredded cheese on the top of the eggs, and fold half the eggs over on top of the other half.

- For an easy, nontraditional cheese omelet: Place 1 ounce of thinly sliced cheese (such as cheddar or Swiss) on top of the eggs. Then, turn the eggs over, and cook an additional 30 seconds. The cheese will be on the bottom of the pan and will become melted and crisp. Flip again so the cheese side is on top before serving.

FRUIT SMOOTHIE

Serves 2

> 1 cup nonfat plain or vanilla kefir (yogurt, soy milk, or almond milk)
>
> 1 large banana
>
> ¼ cup orange juice (or other 100 percent fruit juice)
>
> 1 cup frozen berries (any combination of strawberries, raspberries, blackberries, or blueberries)

1. Place all the ingredients in a blender and purée until smooth. Serve immediately or refrigerate.

Variations

- Try other fruits, such as pineapple, peaches, melons, mango, and papaya, for different taste combinations. Cut the fruit into small pieces before blending.

- On a hot day, add ½ cup crushed ice with the fruit and blend to enjoy a chilled smoothie.

LUNCH

Eating lunch at home? Make sure to save plenty of leftover grilled or roasted vegetables and protein (salmon, chicken, or steak) from the night before, and you'll be able to throw together a quick, neutral meal. Our favorite lunch is leftovers from the night or two before. For a lighter, quicker lunch, we opt for store-bought yogurt with fresh fruit, hummus or baba ghanoush with fresh cut-up vegetables, or low-sodium canned bean soups.

When eating lunch away from home, rethink the usual sandwich option and instead explore fish-of-the-day specials, vegetable and bean (not cream-based) soups, bean-based chilis, lightly dressed salads with some protein, simple grilled chicken, fajitas, or sushi.

BASIC GRILLED CHEESE

Serves 1

> 1–2 ounces cheese (such as American, Cheddar, Swiss, or Havarti)
>
> 2 slices gluten-free bread (lightly toasted, if frozen)
>
> 2–3 teaspoons soft butter

1. Put the cheese between the slices of bread. Spread the top slice of bread with softened butter (or place very thin slices of cold butter over the top of the bread). Season with salt, if desired.

2. Place the sandwich in a small frying pan, butter-side down. Spread more butter on top of the other slice of bread (or place very thin slices of cold butter over the top of it).

3. Cook over medium heat, turning once, until the cheese melts and both sides of the sandwich are golden brown.

QUICK BEEF FAJITAS

Serves 4

4 cloves garlic, minced and mashed into a paste

¼ cup fresh lime juice

2 tablespoons olive oil

1 teaspoon ground cumin

½ teaspoon dried oregano

1 teaspoon freshly ground black pepper

½ teaspoon sea salt

1½ pounds skirt steak, trimmed and cut across the grain diagonally into finger-length strips

Corn tortillas, for serving

Guacamole, for serving

Salsa, for serving

Roasted red peppers, for serving

1. To make the marinade, in a large bowl, whisk together the garlic, lime juice, olive oil, cumin, oregano, pepper, and salt. Add the steak strips and let the meat sit in the marinade for 30 minutes at room temperature.

2. Heat a large, cast-iron skillet over high heat. Remove the meat from the marinade and place it in the hot skillet, working in batches if necessary (do not overcrowd the meat). Cook for 2 minutes, turning the meat every 30 seconds.

3. Serve hot with warm corn tortillas, store-bought guacamole, salsa, and roasted red peppers. Also delicious with rice instead of tortillas.

MEDITERRANEAN LUNCH PLATE

Serves 4

> 4 cups spring salad mix, washed and rinsed
>
> 8 stuffed grape leaves (available jarred, canned, or at a grocery store salad bar)
>
> ½ cup assorted mixed olives
>
> 1 roasted red pepper, thinly sliced (available jarred or roast your own)
>
> 1 cup cubed feta cheese
>
> 1 cup hummus (store-bought from the cheese or deli aisle)
>
> 1 cup baba ghanoush or roasted eggplant spread (store-bought from the cheese or deli aisle)
>
> Olive oil, for drizzling
>
> Assorted gluten-free crackers and breads, for serving
>
> Sugar snap peas, washed and trimmed, for serving

1. Divide the salad mix evenly among 4 dinner-size plates. Place 2 stuffed grape leaves, 4 olives, 4 roasted red pepper slices, and ¼ cup each of the feta, hummus, and baba ghanoush.

2. Drizzle with olive oil, and serve with crackers, bread, and sugar snap peas.

DINNER

The seven dinner menus presented in this chapter (see chart on page 54) are just a sampling of what you'll find in the recipe chapters of this book. We recommend reading through the recipes and finding the ones that will work best for you and your family. You'll also be able to find each of the vegetarian options listed in the index. When you're planning your menus, make your decisions based on the amount of time you'll have to prepare the meal on a given day and the ingredients you'll have on hand—but remember to try to make your meals neutralizing. Visualize your dinner plate and plan to have your alkalizing foods on the left and your acidic foods on the right.

Gluten-Free Good Health Diet Practices

1. Drink 8 ounces of room-temperature water with the juice of half a fresh lemon every day—preferably in the morning, before breakfast.

2. Eat breakfast daily! Your breakfast should provide about 15 percent of your daily calories.

3. Drink green tea and water throughout the day. Use locally sourced honey to sweeten your green tea, if you must. Your beverages, including any alcohol, should equal 10 percent of your daily calories.

4. If you become hungry before lunch, eat a small midmorning snack containing no more than 100 calories.
    Consider the following midmorning snack ideas (perfect for home or office):

    - A piece of fresh fruit, such as an apple or pear
    - Nuts, such as almonds
    - Seeds, such as pumpkin or sunflower
    - A cup of miso soup (conveniently available in a dry form in the Asian section of most grocery stores)

5. Eat a small afternoon snack containing no more than 200 calories, if you are hungry. Consider the following afternoon snack ideas (perfect for home or office):

    - A selection of fresh, cut fruit, such as melon or pineapple
    - Crudités, such as carrot and celery sticks, sugar snap peas, and peppers, paired with your favorite dip
    - Hummus with rice crackers
    - A small sweet treat, such as a cookie, a little chocolate, or a frozen 100 percent fruit bar
    - A small container of yogurt or cottage cheese
    - Any of the midmorning snack ideas

6. It's important to educate yourself about how many calories are in the foods you eat, because if you consume more calories than you need, you'll gain weight. It is that simple.

    To maintain weight: Calories In = Calories Out

    To gain weight: Calories In > Calories Out

    To lose weight: Calories In < Calories Out

It's important for you to realize that even *we* don't count every calorie we eat from day to day—but we did at one time, for a two-week period, in order to learn how many calories our bodies needed. Everyone's needs are different, depending on their size, genetics, and activity levels. Therefore, we recommend that you do the same thing we did: for a two-week period, count all the calories in the food you eat. At the end of each day, record what you have eaten (it's not as easy as you think—remember each mouthful here and bite there) and look up each item's calorie content in a calorie counter (such as *The Complete Book of Food Counts* by Corinne Netzer). Your goal is to have your meals comprise 70 percent of your daily calories: Breakfast should represent 15 percent of the calories, lunch should represent 25 percent, and dinner should represent 30 percent. The breakdowns by meal type for your percentage of daily calories are as follows:

- Breakfast = 15%
- Lunch = 25%
- Dinner = 30%
- Snacks = 15%
- Beverages = 10%
- Goodwill = 5% (your choice to eat or drink a little something extra)

If you prefer to eat four meals a day, replace your snack allocation of 15 percent with a light fourth meal, and space the meals three to four hours apart.

Give yourself a chance to be successful. It takes two full weeks to break your old eating habits, 30 more days to form a new eating pattern, and 90 days for it to become a new lifestyle. Before you start, decide how you will go about breaking your old habits. For instance, when you are offered bread at a restaurant, visualize how you will reward yourself for not eating it—maybe with a delicious piece of dark chocolate.

Don't give up if you slip up. Understand that it is a process, and the process isn't always seamless. Keep at it, and make sure you surround yourself with people and situations that support the healthy lifestyle changes you are trying to make. You may also find it helpful to put your goals into writing. Doing so can make the goals more real and make you feel more accountable.

Remember, there is no miracle food. If there were, everyone would already know about it and be eating it in large quantities. Our ancestors ate a varied seasonal diet, and so should we. The selection and availability of fruits and vegetables in modern supermarkets is incredible. Take the time to explore new foods and tastes, and incorporate the ones you like into meals that balance your health.

REMEMBER THE GLUTEN-FREE GOOD HEALTH DIET PRINCIPLES

1. Test your pH.
2. Eat whole foods.
3. Alkaline foods + acid-forming foods = 0.
4. Go gluten-free.
5. Significantly reduce your intake of sugar and artificial sweeteners.
6. Eliminate diet and regular sodas, and drink more water and green tea.
7. Eat only minimally processed foods, such as frozen plain vegetables and fruits, canned tomatoes, and soup broth.
8. Start each day with fresh lemon water.
9. Learn to cook.
10. Enjoy your food.

CHAPTER 3 REFERENCES

1. Mathews, R. "Importance of Breakfast to Cognitive Performance and Health." *Perspectives in Applied Nutrition* 1996;3(3):204–212.

CHAPTER 4

Getting Started

THE PROCESS OF HOW WE prepare, cook, and eat food has evolved and changed dramatically over the years. In today's culture, few of us hunt or grow much of our own food. Our lives are often filled to the brim with activities, and the process of putting a meal on the table can be left to the last minute—and sometimes, that minute is all we have.

But when it comes to dining in a way that nourishes more than just our bodies—dining that enriches our lives—more than a minute is needed. Cooking is part art and part science. It requires thought, organization, and knowledge, as well as some flair with a skillet. In reality, creativity is nice, but it's not necessary: anyone can follow a recipe. And as is true with most things we set out to do, knowing some basic how-tos in the kitchen can make neutralizing your body much easier.

COOKING: A CRITICAL PART OF CULTURE

Although we are all born with an innate ability to eat, cooking, like many things in life, is something we must learn how to do. Making and eating food is part of every known culture on earth. In fact, according to Dr. Richard W. Wrangham, a professor of anthropology at Harvard University, preparing food and eating it in a social setting are so central to the human experience that the culinary arts may well be what made us human in the first place. He explained, "There's no record anywhere of any people who have lived without cooking." (*New York Times*, May 28, 2002)

We believe home-cooked meals made with high-quality, fresh foods are essential for a neutralized body and a balanced life. In the time you might otherwise spend watching 30 minutes of reality TV, you could prepare a meal that brings your family together and satisfies body, mind, and soul. The act of preparing fresh food, of chopping and sautéing, provides mental stimulation and grounds us in the salt-and-pepper realities of everyday life. It is a small but important way to give meaning to the abstraction of daily living. We

DOING FOR ONESELF

My first real sense of doing for oneself came about during the summer of my 18th year, when I found myself lost in the wilds of Idaho. I had taken a job as a USDA forest ranger for the summer. My job was to watch for forest fires from a tower perched high on a mountain, eight miles from the nearest road. The tower was so remote that I was flown by helicopter to the top of the mountain with my supplies for the entire summer.

I had been on the job for only ten days when I had got my first four-day break. What was supposed to be a three-hour hike down the mountain turned into 32 hours of survival training. I got disoriented in a snow-covered valley, and my government-issue compass's magnetic north was off by several degrees. I went the wrong way, and by the time I realized my mistake, I was deep into the forest. To protect myself against hypothermia that night, I dug a hole, climbed inside, and covered myself with leaves. In the morning, I decided to try to regain some of my strength and stamina by napping on a sunny boulder—only to be awakened by a curious moose.

I knew the safest way out was to follow the meandering river, which would eventually wind past a campsite. I bushwhacked my way through virgin lands, retracing the footsteps of Lewis and Clark. Twenty-six hours into my ordeal, a rescue helicopter flew directly over me. After screaming and throwing my backpack wildly into the air—all to no avail—I knew the only thing I could trust was my own instinct, faith, and abilities. After a good cry, I picked myself up and walked for another six hours straight until I found a campground.

There, some kind campers took me under their wing and offered me a hot meal of pork chops, applesauce, and a couple of shots of Jack Daniel's. It warmed my body and nourished my soul—the ultimate in comfort food. That simple, delicious meal is forever embedded in my memory. I can still smell the campfire, visualize the paper plate brimming with food, taste the juicy pork chops, and feel the whiskey burn my throat.

Decades later, whenever I reflect back on the experience, I think about two things. Doing for oneself gives you confidence and self-worth, and food, even in its most basic form, can bring lasting memories and meaning to one's life. Somehow over the years the two things have become one, and today, the simple act of planning and cooking a meal fills me with meaning.   —*Claudia Pillow*

believe that all those highly processed, powdered, and dehydrated chemical food products—many of which contain gluten—are robbing us of nutrition, flavor, and the chance to nurture our most basic needs. Thus, doing for oneself (and for others) should not be underestimated.

Our basic how-to is actually a system that can be used for any type of cooking you do, whether it's a simple everyday meal or a multicourse dinner party.

PLAN AND SHOP

We think of dinner as something to relax with and enjoy. No rushing is allowed. It should be something to look forward to, a nice ending to the work or school day, or a special evening with friends. We like to make foods that we can anticipate eating with pleasure.

Naturally, there are times when commitments (sports, activities, meetings, work, and so forth) get in the way of these dinners. But that makes it all the more important to dine well when we can. And yes, there are many occasions when high-quality convenience foods can save you a lot of preparation time. (There's nothing like a jarred pasta sauce you didn't have to simmer for hours on a busy night.) In fact, some of our recipes include or recommend prepared convenience food products we like and use all the time.

But with or without the inclusion of ready-made foods in the meal, timing is just as important as the menu and ingredients. How and when you prep, cook, and serve matters. Bad timing can destroy good food. Like playing a sport, pulling together a delicious dinner and serving it in a relaxed environment requires careful thought, effort, and practice.

We strive to make each meal special but achievable by following these simple steps:

- **Think carefully about when you will be eating at home during the week and with whom**. Who in the household has to be where at what time? Any special occasions? Dinner parties? How many everyday meals will you be preparing for the week, and what are the time constraints for each? Which meals have to be quick, and which can be leisurely?

- **Consider what you really want to eat over the course of the week for those everyday meals**. Is it cold enough outside for stew? Do you feel like grilling? Have you been craving Mexican? Will you be dining out at all this week, or at friends' homes? Do you need to plan meals that are on the lighter side? Are there any special requests from people you will be eating with? Try not to overreach.

- **Loosely organize the menus in your mind or on paper, if necessary**. When possible, check your calendar for the upcoming week during the weekend, when you have more time to prepare. That's an ideal time to map out meals for at least the first few days of the week. The leftovers from Sunday's stew could be great for a dinner after a busy Monday. Maybe the kids' favorite, barbecued chicken, would be a good fit for Tuesday. You might want to try out a new fish recipe on Wednesday, and perhaps dine out on Thursday. This simple step of menu planning will enable you to better control what and how you eat each day. It can also help reduce food waste and increase time efficiency.

- **Make a shopping list**. Focus on the main dish for each meal and how you plan to cook it. What ingredients will you need? You may want to plan your side dishes around what looks fresh and good at the store, or what's on sale. Consider what foods you have in the house, and what you need to buy. In order to cook delicious meals, it helps to have a well-stocked pantry full of foods you can turn to at a moment's notice. See our pantry suggestions at the end of this chapter for some ideas. A very quick shopping trip may be necessary on Saturday or Sunday to provide ingredients for weekend dinners and the beginning of the week. But you can avoid the weekend crunch at the store and achieve the same results by making the trip on Friday or Monday. It's best to focus your shopping in the outer perimeter of the grocery store (produce, dairy, and the meat and seafood counters) and avoid the center aisles of the store, where most processed foods (and most shoppers) are located. You may also want to visit a local specialty market. Midweek is usually the least busy time at the supermarkets, so if you can, save your trips to the store's inside aisles for an off-peak visit

- **Give a little thought ahead of time about how and when you will make each meal**. Which meals can be prepped or even cooked ahead? How can leftovers be used (if there are any)?

- **Last, try to practice**. Take chances. Expect a few failures. Subscribe to a food magazine. Try something new. All the while, keep your focus on building a repertoire of dependable, delicious foods you can look forward to making and eating.

How well you cook depends on how well you shop. Try to buy locally grown foods in season and shop for real food of high quality. So how do you know what a real food is? Well, if an eight-year-old can't tell what the original form of the food was, you probably shouldn't be eating it. This down-and-dirty method works well for meat, poultry, fish, fruits, vegetables, beans, nuts, whole grains, and dairy—the foods that should make up the core of your diet. These are the "real foods" you find at farmers markets, many specialty shops, and on the outer aisles of the grocery store. On the outside aisles of the supermarket, you will find ingredients in their original forms. These are foods you may have to do more with than simply heat them up, but they are foods that will ultimately satisfy more of your real needs.

PREP AND SERVE

When it comes to prepping, cooking, and serving a meal, it helps to be organized if you want to do it well. Figure out approximately how long the meal will take to put together. Allow yourself enough time so you aren't in a frenzied state by the time you sit down to eat. This is where practice and having a repertoire of recipes you know how to cook can make your life easier. Here are a few simple things to remember:

- **Clean up as you go along.** This is a critical, but often overlooked, necessity for a relaxed meal. It's far more pleasant to eat in a kitchen that doesn't look like a daunting wasteland of dirty dishes (even by candlelight, piles of dishes loom large). It also reduces the cleanup time after dinner, when you'll probably want to relax.

- **Start with the most time-consuming dish first.** Take out all the ingredients, and prep as much as possible before you start to cook the dish. If the item is something that has to cook for a while, you can finish the side dishes after you get it started. If it's something that has to be finished at the last minute, prep it up to the finishing point, and then get the sides ready.

- **Many side dishes can be prepped and cooked a little ahead of time and then simply reheated in a microwave as the main dish finishes cooking.** This also makes for a lighter cleanup after the meal, because some of the pots can be washed and put away ahead of time.

- **Some evenings, we finish cooking a main dish that has been already been prepped (or cooked up to the point where it can be simply finished) after eating the meal's first course, a salad.** This gives us additional time with our families or dining companions to talk about the day as they sit at the table. It also stretches out the meal and allows our bodies time to begin to digest some of the first course before beginning the next; we've found that it helps prevent overeating later in the meal (it takes about 20 minutes for your body to register the feeling of food filling your stomach).

- **Take an extra moment of time to make the plates or serving dishes of food look appealing to the eye.** Arrange the food in an attractive way. When possible, use a garnish to give the dish extra color, flavor, or interest.

- **Finally, try to create a more relaxed backdrop for your dinner by setting the mood.** Make the table look pretty. Play some quiet music. Dim the overhead light fixtures, and maybe light a few candles. (Even rambunctious children have been known to respond in a positive way to a calmer, less brightly lit environment.) Mentally leave your problems behind and enjoy the moment. Make it seem special even though it's only Tuesday and you're just enjoying some simple chili. Strive, with enthusiasm and practice to make all your dinners special.

BASIC COOKING METHODS

The Science of Roasting

Traditional roasting. Roasting is a method of dry-heat cooking that uses minimal liquid in an uncovered pan in the oven. It produces a well-browned, caramelized exterior and, ideally, a moist, succulent interior. Roasting requires reasonably tender pieces of beef, lamb, or pork usually placed on a rack, fat-side up, so the fat bastes the meat as it melts. In addition to these red meat options, any kind of poultry and most fish are also well suited to roasting.

High-heat roasting. This method is often preferred for beef and pork tenderloins, beef and pork top loin cuts, some fish, and some small, unstuffed whole poultry. In this preparation, the meat is roasted at a high temperature until it is cooked to the desired temperature.

Searing. This method combines high and moderate heat. The meat or poultry is first cooked in a very hot (usually 450°F) oven to sear the exterior and then roasted slowly at a lower temperature (usually 325°F). As a result, the meat forms a crusty exterior and a tender interior. The searing method is used for meat that is well marbled with fat to help keep it from drying out (such as a rib roast) and large whole poultry.

Slow roasting. A slow-roasting method is used for tougher cuts of meat that are less marbled with fat (for example, top round roasts or beef sirloin roasts). Since the meat has less fat to keep it moist, it is cooked at a lower temperature, usually 325°–350°F, in order to keep it from drying out. Slow roasting is also used for meats that are very fatty, because the long, slow cooking allows the fat to soften and melt off, leaving behind tender, juicy meat.

Broiling. Broiling is roasting at a very high temperature next to the heat source. It is good for particularly tender cuts of meat that are on the smallish side (for example, burgers, steaks, chops, fish, and smaller pieces of poultry), because the meat will cook for only a short time. The broiler should be preheated.

Below is our classic roasting technique, in five basic steps:

1. **Remove your meat, poultry, or fish from the refrigerator** about an hour before roasting to allow it to come close to room temperature and soften up a bit. If it has been resting in a marinade or brine, pat it dry. Following these steps will facilitate even cooking.

2. **Season your meat, poultry, or fish** before roasting with salt, pepper, and other spices or herbs, if desired. If you are using a rub or paste, follow the recipe. This step will enhance and deepen your meat's natural flavors.

3. **Roast your meat, poultry, or fish using the appropriate heat method** until it is cooked to the desired internal temperature or degree of doneness. Smaller pieces

(less than 2 pounds) of beef, pork, or lamb should be browned in a hot skillet on the stovetop before roasting, because they will not have enough time to brown in the oven.

4. **Remove the meat or poultry from the oven just before it's fully cooked** because the meat's internal temperature will continue to rise by 5° to 10°F as the meat rests.

5. **Allow meat, poultry, and whole fish to rest after roasting for at least 10 minutes** (more for larger roasts) so the fibers in the meat can relax. The juices, which expand during the meat's time in the oven, shrink as the food cools. A resting period permits the juices to flow back through the fibers. Your meat will be more moist and firm and easier to carve.

The Science of Grilling

We like to use gas grills because they are easy to start, easy to control, and easy to clean. Yes, we love smokers, and yes, we love the taste of charcoal-grilled food, but we consider gas grilling an everyday cooking method, not just something we save for a leisurely Sunday afternoon. We grill year-round—in the sun, rain, and snow—because it is as effortless as turning on the oven.

Direct-heat grilling. This method of grilling involves cooking food directly over the heat source at a high temperature until it is cooked to the desired internal temperature or degree of doneness. It is used for foods that are tender, not too thick, and can be cooked quickly, such as beef, lamb, and pork tenderloins; some steaks; hamburgers; hot dogs; sausages; fish; vegetables; and kabobs of all sizes.

Indirect-heat grilling. Indirect-heat grilling combines high and moderate heat. The meat is first seared quickly over hot, direct heat and then moved to a part of the grilling rack away from the grill's flame (with a gas grill, the burner under the food should be turned off and the remaining burners should be turned down to 275° to 325° F). It is used for larger pieces of meat, roasts and whole poultry, or for meat that needs to be cooked slowly, such as a rack of ribs.

THE TOUCH METHOD

The "touch method" of testing for doneness means to compare how the meat feels to the firmness of your hand using a quick touch with your index finger. Well done feels firm, like the ball of your thumb; rare feels soft, like the fleshy part between your thumb and index finger; and medium is somewhere in between.

These grilling basics will ensure perfectly grilled foods:

1. **Remove your meat, poultry, or fish from the refrigerator** about an hour before grilling to allow it to come close to room temperature and soften up a bit. If it has been resting in a marinade or brine, pat it dry. Following these steps will facilitate even cooking.

2. **Season your meat, poultry, or fish before grilling** with salt, pepper, and other spices or herbs, if desired. If you are using a rub or paste, follow the recipe. This step will enhance and deepen your meat's natural flavors.

3. **Make sure your grill is clean before you start cooking.** Cleaning the grill helps prevent flare-ups, which can burn the meat.

4. **Preheat the grill according to your recipe.** Doing so will help sear the outside of the meat and prevent it from drying out.

5. **Lightly oil the grill rack before cooking** in order to prevent the food from sticking.

6. **Use cooking tongs to turn your food only when necessary.** Doing so allows the meat to brown and caramelize without losing too many juices.

7. **Remove the food from the grill just before it is completely cooked** because the meat's internal temperature will continue to rise by 5° to 10°F as the meat rests. Exact grill times are difficult to predict due to variable factors, so test for doneness a few minutes before the recommended cook time. Touch the meat to measure its doneness or use a meat thermometer when necessary (especially for larger pieces).

8. **Allow meat, poultry, and fish to rest after grilling** for at least 5 minutes for smaller pieces (burgers, fish fillets, and so on), and 10 minutes for larger pieces so the fibers in the meat can relax. The juices, which expand during the meat's time on the grill, shrink as the food cools. A resting period permits the juices to flow back through the fibers. Your meat will be more moist and firm, and easier to carve.

The Science of Sautéing

Sautéing or pan-frying is a great way to get dinner on the table fast. In this method, tender, single-size portions of meat, poultry, or fish are cooked in a small amount of oil or another fat in a skillet or sauté pan over direct heat. The food is not submerged in fat as with deep-frying. Pans for sautéing should be hot enough for the food to sizzle, but the fat and meat should not smoke. It is important to ensure that the food is dry before placing it in a hot pan and that the pan stays hot throughout the cooking process.

After the meat, poultry, or fish is sautéed, it is removed from the pan to a nearby dish and tented with foil. The hot pan is deglazed by adding a small amount of liquid (usually stock, wine, or vinegar) and stirring to loosen browned bits of food from the bottom. The result is the basis for a quick pan sauce.

A solid, deep-sided frying pan (or skillet) is an invaluable piece of kitchen equipment. We use an assortment of inexpensive nonstick (6-, 10-, and 12-inch diameter pans that are 1 to 2 inches deep) and heavy-grade (12-inch diameter and 2 inches deep, with a tight-fitting lid) skillets and frying pans.

Following is our basic sauté method in five steps:

1. **Sauté**. Prepare the meat, poultry, or seafood according to the recipe. Heat the oil and/or butter in a heavy skillet over medium-high to high heat. Add the meat and cook, without moving the meat, until the underside is brown. Turn the meat over to brown the other side. Don't crowd the pan, or the food will steam instead of brown.

2. **Flavor**. Remove the meat to a platter, tent it with foil, and set it aside. Add an aromatic or vegetable—garlic, shallots, onions, and/or mushrooms—to the pan and sauté until soft, about 2 minutes.

3. **Deglaze**. Add broth, wine, or vinegar to the pan and scrape loose any browned bits stuck to the bottom of the pan.

4. **Reduce**. Add any remaining sauce ingredients (such as tomatoes, cream, and/or seasonings) and bring to a boil, stirring frequently, for the desired time or according to the recipe directions. Boiling will reduce and thicken your sauce and create deeper flavors.

5. **Serve**. Return the meat to the pan containing the sauce. You may either cook the meat with the sauce for a brief amount of time (to rewarm it and evenly distribute the sauce) or simply pour the sauce over the meat and serve immediately.

The Science of Braising and Stewing

Braising, a good choice for tough cuts of meat and some sturdy vegetables, involves browning food in fat and then cooking it, tightly covered, on the stovetop in a small amount of liquid at a low heat for a long period of time. This long, slow cooking develops flavor and tenderizes foods by gently breaking down their fibers.

Stewing is a moist-heat cooking method on the stovetop in which smaller pieces of meat or poultry are barely covered with liquid and simmered for a long period of time in a tightly covered pot. Stewing not only tenderizes tough pieces of meat but also allows the flavors of the ingredients to blend deliciously.

Following is our classic braising and stewing technique in six basic steps:

1. **Remove your meat or poultry from the refrigerator** about an hour before braising or stewing to allow it to come close to room temperature and soften up a bit. If it has been resting in a marinade or brine (for example, corned beef), pat it dry. Following these steps will facilitate even cooking.

2. **Season your meat or poultry before braising or stewing** with salt, pepper, and other spices or herbs, if desired. This step will enhance and deepen your meat's natural flavors.

3. **Brown the meat or poultry in very hot oil** on the stovetop in a Dutch oven or another type of heavy-bottomed pot with a tight-fitting lid. For stews, it may be necessary to divide cubed meat into smaller batches so it browns quickly without beginning to cook. (If your stew recipe calls for the meat to be floured use plain brown rice flour for a gluten-free version.) Browning will help give the dish a boost in color and flavor.

4. **Remove the meat or poultry from the pot and add any vegetables and/or aromatics** (usually some combination of onion, carrots, celery, garlic, or shallots) that will be used to flavor the dish. Sauté the vegetables in the fat and juices left in the pot until softened. Spices can also be added at this stage.

5. **Add any liquids** (usually some combination of stock and wine) to the pot and scrape up any brown bits left in the bottom. Return the meat to the pot and add any other seasonings, including other vegetables and fresh herbs. Bring to a simmer. Reduce the heat to low, cover the pot, and cook until the meat or poultry is tender (or you can also finish cooking it in the oven at a very low heat). Additional vegetables (carrots, potatoes, and so on) can be added about 1 to 1½ hours before the meat or poultry is finished.

6. **Remove the meat or poultry and vegetables and boil the liquid** on the stovetop until it reaches the desired thickness. (Some or all of the vegetables can be puréed and added to the juices to further thicken and flavor the mixture.)

A Few More Techniques

- **"Bring to a boil"** means to heat a liquid until bubbles break the surface (212°F for water at sea level). To "boil" means to cook food in a boiling liquid.

- **Simmer** and poach mean to cook food gently in liquid at a temperature low enough (usually around 185°F) that tiny bubbles just begin to break the surface.

- **Steam** means to cook food by placing it on a rack or in a special steamer basket over water that is boiling or simmering in a covered pan. Steaming is a more effective method than boiling or poaching for retaining a food's flavor, shape, texture, and many of its nutrients.

- **Caramelize** means to expose food to heat in order to liquefy and then brown its natural sugars. By browning the sugars, you help develop the food's flavor and enhance its aroma. Technically, to "caramelize" means to cook sugar, but over the years, use of the term has expanded. You will often find instructions to "caramelize onions," for example, in order to make them taste sweeter.

RECOMMENDED COOKING TEMPERATURES

Heating meat and poultry to the right temperature destroys harmful microorganisms, but at the same time, we find that it's important to take our meat and poultry off the heat a little bit before it is completely done in order to allow it to "rest." It will continue to cook as it stands, which is why we take it off a bit early. The meat's flavorful juices expand during cooking, and then shrink and get redistributed throughout the meat as it cools. It becomes juicier and easier to slice.

We remove meat from the heat source when it reaches the temperatures listed below and then allow it to rest for 5 to 15 minutes (depending on weight). Allow larger pieces to rest longer.

	Fahrenheit	Celsius
Beef/Lamb/Veal		
Rare	125–130°F	51–54°C
Medium	135–140°F	57–60°C
Well done	155°F	68°C
Pork `	155°F	68°C
Chicken and Turkey*	170°F	76°C
Fish	120 to 137°F	49 to 58°C
Ground Meats		
Beef, lamb, veal, pork	160°F	71°C
Chicken, turkey	165°F	74°C

* Determine temperature by inserting an instant-read thermometer between thigh and breast

HERBS

To replace dried herbs with fresh herbs in a recipe, use a 1:3 proportion—for every 1 teaspoon of dried herbs, use 3 teaspoons (or 1 tablespoon) of chopped fresh herbs. If you are cooking a dish for more than 20 minutes and you are substituting fresh herbs for dried in the recipe, we recommend you add about half the total amount when called for in the recipe. Then, you should wait until the dish is almost ready (about 10 minutes before serving) to add the remaining half in order to avoid cooking out the flavors. For cold dishes, such as bean salads, add either dried or fresh herbs several hours in advance to give the flavors a chance to meld.

THE ART OF COOKING

Some people need to follow recipes exactly as written. Other people read a recipe, close the book, and start cooking. If you are like most people, you're somewhere in between. Your level of confidence, experience, and creativity will define what you do with any given set of directions. But food varies in quality, form, taste, and smell. The type of pan it is cooked in varies from home to home. There's no such thing as a foolproof recipe. So how do *you* use the recipes in the *Gluten-Free Good Health Cookbook*?

This book assumes you understand basic culinary terms, such as chopping, dicing, beating, and so on. It also assumes you have a well-stocked pantry. If you are relatively new to cooking, follow these recipes closely, but use your own judgment. Taste, touch, and smell the food often as you cook it. If a recipe says that you should sauté for 4 minutes but it looks done after 2 minutes, trust your senses and move on to the next step.

DAIRY AND EGG REPLACEMENTS

Egg substitutes: You can use ¼ cup of whipped silken tofu to replace a large egg in many recipes, especially bread. In addition, Ener-G-Replacer and another homemade remedy (1½ tablespoons water, 1½ tablespoons canola oil, and 1½ teaspoons baking powder) can produce a good, but not always ideal, result in some recipes.

Milk substitutes: Rice, soy, and almond milk can be used to replace cow's milk. Rice and almond milk have less of an aftertaste, unless you like the taste of soy.

Butter substitutes: Smart Balance is a good substitute for butter in baking and cooking. Use higher-fat versions (64 percent or higher).

After you have completed the cooking process, taste the food again. Note any changes you've made to the recipe—or that you want to make to it—right on the page so you'll have a record of it for next time around. There—you're on your way to building your own repertoire of recipes.

If you are an experienced cook, use these recipes as a guide. Adjust the seasonings and ingredients to your tastes, but follow the basic cooking procedures and techniques. Cooking times and temperatures may vary and the amounts of ingredients may change, but the preparation method should be consistent.

Artful Ways to Add Variety to Your Food

Marinades are used to make meats, fish, and vegetables extra flavorful, moist, and tender. They are composed of three key elements: acids to tenderize (usually wine, vinegar, citrus juice, soy sauce, buttermilk, or yogurt), oils to moisten, and herbs and spices to flavor. Sugars (including brown sugar, honey, and molasses) are often used to balance the acid and enhance browning. Food is typically soaked in a marinade anywhere from 30 minutes (for fish) to overnight (for meats and poultry). Poultry and fish will begin to toughen and turn white if it is left for too long in an acidic marinade.

Rubs are combinations of herbs and spices applied directly to the skin or flesh of meat, poultry, and fish. Rubs are typically spread over meats and poultry anywhere from an hour before cooking to overnight, and over fish about an hour before cooking.

Pastes are a combination of herbs and spices with a small amount of liquid, usually oil or a touch of soy sauce or citrus juice. Like rubs, they are applied directly to the skin or flesh of meat, poultry, and fish. Like rubs, pastes are typically spread over meats and poultry anywhere from an hour before cooking to overnight, and over fish about an hour before cooking.

Brines are salt solutions that are often flavored with herbs, spices, sugars, and other flavorings. They are used to tenderize and flavor meat and poultry. Meat and poultry are soaked in brine solutions for anywhere from 8 hours to 2 days before cooking.

By using a small variety of ingredients, you can substantially alter the flavor and character of your foods. In this book, we've offered up many of our favorite recipes, the ones we make all the time. You can make them as is, or by altering the herbs, spices, oils, or acids, you can fine-tune them to your own liking. We offer suggestions for variations at the end of many recipes.

PANTRY SUGGESTIONS

We recommend that you read food labels carefully if you want or need to avoid gluten. It is a hidden ingredient in many foods, including soy sauce, broth, malt vinegars, condiments, and cereal (usually in the form of barley malt flavoring). Oatmeal is often contaminated with gluten, but there are excellent uncontaminated versions available in stores that are clearly labeled "gluten free." (In addition, many people with gluten sensitivity also consider oatmeal that comes from Ireland and Finland to be safe.)

Nonrefrigerated*

Red wine vinegar

White distilled vinegar

Rice wine vinegar

Apple cider vinegar

Balsamic vinegar

Canola oil

Extra virgin olive oil

Walnut oil

Sesame oil

Hot and spicy oil

Worcestershire sauce

Tamari soy sauce

Hoisin sauce

Fish sauce

Red and white wine

Sherry, Port, and Marsala wine

Rice wine or sake

Honey

Molasses

Maple syrup

Favorite bottled barbecue sauce

Favorite bottled salad dressing (we use Newman's Own Olive Oil & Vinegar Dressing as a quick marinade)

Ketchup

Mayonnaise

Assorted mustards

Favorite bottled salsas

Canned whole tomatoes

Canned diced tomatoes

Canned crushed tomatoes

Canned tomato paste

Jars of your favorite pasta sauce

Canned red kidney, black, and cannellini beans

Assorted favorite relishes and pickles

Brine-cured olives and oil-cured olives

Capers

Assorted fruit preserves

* Many of these items require refrigeration after opening. Check the labels to be sure.

Assorted favorite rice crackers

Assorted dried fruits (raisins, apricots, currants, etc.)

Fresh garlic

Onions

Shallots

Ginger

Long-grain white rice

Brown rice

Arborio rice

Basmati rice

Assorted dried pasta (we recommend Tinkyada and Schaar brands)

Asian rice noodles

Assorted dry beans

Iodized salt

Sea salt

Kosher salt

Whole black peppercorns

Whole mixed peppercorns

Freshly ground black pepper

A variety of dried herbs and spices, including: allspice, basil, bay leaf, cardamom, cayenne pepper, cinnamon, assorted chili powders, Chinese five-spice powder, whole cloves, ground cloves, coriander, crushed red pepper, cumin seeds, ground cumin, curry powder, dill weed, fennel seed, dried mustard, ground ginger, nutmeg, oregano, paprika, red pepper flakes, rosemary, sage, saffron, tarragon, thyme leaves, ground thyme, and turmeric (just to name a few)

Beef, veal, and chicken glace and/or demi-glace (we recommend More than Gourmet brand)

Concentrated fish glace (we recommend More than Gourmet brand)

Bottled clam juice

Cans or boxes of low-sodium chicken, beef, and/or vegetable broth

Millet flour

Sorghum flour

Potato starch (not potato flour)

Tapioca flour (also called tapioca starch)

Cornstarch

Xanthan gum

Stone-ground corn meal

Extra-finely ground brown rice flour*

Sweet rice flour (preferably extra finely ground)*

Granulated sugar

Dark brown sugar

Buckwheat flour

Powdered buttermilk

* A recommended source for gluten-free extra finely ground brown rice flour and sweet rice flour: Authentic Foods, 1860 W. 169th St., Suite B, Gardena, CA 90247
Phone: 800-806-4737 or 310-366-7612. Web site: www.authenticfoods.com

Refrigerated

Butter

Heavy cream

Eggs

Milk

Sour cream (or high-quality reduced-fat sour cream)

Aged Parmigiano-Reggiano cheese

Other assorted cheeses (Montrachet, cheddar, Monterey Jack)

Carrots

Celery

Lemons and limes (grated zest can be stored in the freezer)

Bacon and pancetta (or wrap into individual portions and store in freezer for soups, stews, and bean dishes)

Prepared pesto (can also be stored in freezer)

Bottled minced garlic

Assorted nuts (walnuts, almonds, and pecans)

Assorted fresh herbs you use often

What's to Come?

The *Gluten-Free Good Health Cookbook* is a distinct departure from other diet cookbooks. Our focus is on teaching you how to manage daily food-related decisions in order to strengthen your immune system, prevent disease, and lose weight—all while eating real food. We conceived of it as part science-based diet book and part cookbook. We provide food choice explanations and guidance, cooking advice, and flavorful, culturally diverse recipes. But unlike most diet books, we include cooking instruction as well: We've combined the science of diet books with the culinary techniques you find in classic cookbooks.

Therefore, we start the recipe portion of the book with Chapter 5: Sauces and Gravies, which are the cornerstones of all kinds of delicious meals. Included are more than a dozen innovative recipes for sauce and soup bases and traditional gravies that use puréed vegetables to thicken and enhance flavor in lieu of flour and fats. More traditional recipes for gluten-free Roux and Classic Cheese Sauce are included at the end of the chapter.

The rest of the book is laid out like a classic cookbook. Soup, chowders, and chili recipes are showcased in Chapter 6. We zero in on the art and science of making good-tasting vegetables in Chapter 7. Chapter 8 contains deliciously gluten-free, grain-based recipes. A rich variety of fish, poultry, and meat recipes are detailed in Chapters 9 through 11, and Chapter 12 features 12 delightful desserts—many of which do not involve baking. These are the recipes we make every day in our own homes, the ones that our families and friends look forward to, and the ones we count on to help us make mealtimes both healthy and happy. We hope they will inspire you to cook and develop your own repertoire of tried and true stress-free recipes.

CHAPTER 5

Sauces and Gravies
Creating Your Own Convenience Foods

UNLESS THERE IS A SEISMIC SHIFT in the way food is produced and sold in this country, it will be a decade before it is no longer a challenge to buy ready-made foods for those who follow a gluten-free diet. In the meantime, many high-quality convenience foods are naturally gluten-free and can easily be incorporated into a meal—pasta sauces, salsas, canned tomatoes, broths, certain brands of flash-frozen fruits and vegetables, and dried gluten-free pastas need only to be enhanced with other ingredients to create delicious, healthy dishes.

Conversely, another group of highly processed convenience foods—sauces, gravies, and soups—are unavailable to people on a gluten-free diet, because most boxes, cans, and bags of these highly processed foods contain gluten. But perhaps that's for the best: These foods are also highly acidic to the body because they contain sugar (often in the form of high-fructose corn syrup), salt, fats, and various other chemicals that enhance their flavor and extend their shelf life. We shouldn't be eating this food in the first place, but we still crave mashed potatoes and gravy, pot pies, and macaroni and cheese every once in a while for dinner. So get out your saucepan and some gluten-free broth, and let's get started.

Introduction to Creamy Sauce Bases

Creamy Chicken Sauce Base

   Creamy Chicken Garlic Sauce Base

Creamy Beef Sauce Base

   Creamy Beef Garlic Sauce Base

Creamy Mushroom Sauce Base for Gravy and Soup

   Creamy Mushroom Garlic Sauce Base

Introduction to Creamy Soup Bases

Creamy Chicken Soup Base

Creamy Beef Soup Base

Old-Fashioned Saucepan Chicken Gravy

Old-Fashioned Saucepan Beef Gravy

Old-Fashioned Saucepan Mushroom Gravy

Roux

Cheese Sauce

THE SCIENCE OF CREATING GLUTEN-FREE SAUCES AND GRAVIES

Professional chefs have the time and staff to make rich, flavorful stocks and demi-glaces. Simmering pots of caramelized vegetables and bones that have been slow-roasted for hours are used to make soups, stews, sauces, quick sautés, gravies, risottos, and even pasta dishes. Homemade stock and demi-glace in a recipe can make the difference between extraordinary and everyday, but it's not always possible. Maintaining a gluten-free lifestyle can be time consuming enough, but having to stay home to simmer a veal stock for eight hours (good news: it's only five hours for beef!) could put you over the edge.

What is the difference between stock and broth? Stock is usually the more substantial of the two. It is made by cooking bones, meat trimmings, water, and diced vegetables (in classic French cooking, the diced combination of vegetables is called a mirepoix—carrots, celery, and onions) for a very long time. Stock is used as a base for soups, stews, sauces, and many other dishes.

Broth is usually lighter and less substantial. It is made from meat, water, and vegetables and is cooked for a shorter period of time. Broth can be used just as it is to make a soup enhanced with meat, rice, noodles, and vegetables, or it can be used in place of stock in a variety of other dishes.

What are glaces and demi-glaces? A glace is flavorful, reduced stock. A demi-glace is a sauce made from stock, a roux (a cooked mixture of butter and flour; see our gluten-free versions on page 96), caramelized vegetables, herbs, and sometimes wine and tomato paste. It has a very concentrated flavor and is used to enhance sauces, sautés, stews, and soups.

When time is in short supply, good-quality store-bought broths can be enhanced and made more substantial by adding caramelized vegetables, herbs, and spices. In addition, high-quality gluten-free demi-glace products are available in grocery stores around the country and online (see our recommendation on the next page). We make liberal use of both in this book, although we happily substitute homemade whenever it is available.

Our focus here is to provide a variety of flavorful sauce and soup bases that can be used to create delicious meals, in much the same way processed foods made with gluten are often incorporated into recipes. The bases all start with purchased or homemade stock or broth, although we do not provide instructions to make homemade stock—because there are so many good ones already in print. Julia Child, Marcella Hazan, Patricia Wells, the *Gourmet Cookbook*, and many other sources all provide well-balanced and naturally gluten-free stock recipes.

Our bases put classic cooking techniques to work in three basic steps:

1. **Sauté and caramelize** some combination of onions, shallots, leeks, garlic, carrots and celery in a tiny bit of oil. The purpose of this step is to help the base develop a richer, more complex flavor.

2. Add the stock/broth to **deglaze** the pan (that means you scrape up the brown caramelized bits that remain stuck to the pan and simmer until the mixture is reduced. The purpose is to concentrate the flavors.

3. **Purée** the stock/broth and the vegetable mixture to create a creamy, flavorful base. This base can be used as is or enhanced with additional broth, cream, or wine (including Port).

THE ART OF CREATING GLUTEN-FREE SAUCES AND GRAVIES

These bases use few ingredients, but by varying the ingredients—beef broth instead of chicken broth, leeks instead of onions, or shallots instead of garlic—or by adding herbs, spices, wine, or cream, you can create a number of delicious variations. We give suggestions and ideas so you will be able to see how each base can be used in a variety of dishes. We want you think of each recipe as a starting point for your own tastes and creativity.

Make several different kinds in large batches and keep them in ready-to-use–sized containers in the freezer. Reach for one to enhance a quick sauté or create a savory stew or a creamy soup. We usually depend on puréed vegetables to add complexity and thickness, but you can add cream, if desired. Once you have a variety of bases stocked in your freezer, you'll be able to make flavorful gravies and sauces without much of the preparation typically required.

Demi-glace, Reduced Sauces (Glaces), and Reduced Stock

It's almost impossible to find prepared classic demi-glace made without wheat flour. Although we embrace the idea of homemade everything, we know we'll probably never be able to set aside the enormous amount of time it takes to make one in our own kitchens. Luckily, More Than Gourmet makes a delicious assortment of high-quality concentrated stocks and glaces that we happily use. All of their stocks and glaces, except their classic veal demi-glace, are gluten free. They are sold in grocery stores and by online retailers such as Amazon.com. Contact More Than Gourmet at (800) 860-9389 or www.morethangourmet.com.

INTRODUCTION TO MAKING CREAMY SAUCE BASES

These flavorful sauce bases will come in handy for making gravies, sautés, gratins, and casseroles. Infuse them with any combination of herbs and spices to create a rich variety of classic dishes from cuisines around the world. You can use them as a cooking sauce for recipes made on the stove or in the oven. They are complex enough to stand alone, but so simple that their character can be changed by the addition of a touch of cream or spice. They are rich enough to serve as a nearly fat-free alternative to cream- or roux-based sauces. In short, they will become a reliable ingredient in your cooking repertoire.

Take note: A vegetarian version can be made with low-sodium vegetable broth. Just follow the instructions for the Creamy Chicken Sauce Base, but use vegetable broth in place of chicken broth.

Ideas for how to use the creamy sauce bases:

- Add the herb-infused Creamy Chicken Sauce with a dash of wine and cream to top off a quick sauté of chicken cutlets.

- Use the herb-infused Creamy Beef Sauce as a flavorful base for beef stew (along with some red wine). Add potatoes, mushrooms, baby onions, peas, and carrots toward the end of the cooking time.

- Mix the Creamy Chicken Garlic Sauce with a bit of cream and grated cheese to make a chicken noodle gratin (see page 169).

- Add a dash of cognac and cream to the Creamy Beef Sauce to top off a steak au poivre.

- Purée the Creamy Chicken Sauce with canned or freshly roasted chopped green chilies to top an enticing casserole made with shredded chicken, cheese, and corn tortillas (see page 218).

- Mix the herb-infused Creamy Beef Sauce with a touch of red wine to make a sauce for savory braised short ribs.

- Mix the Creamy Beef Sauce with sour cream and sautéed mushrooms to make a quick beef Stroganoff.

- Make the Creamy Chicken Garlic Sauce with Chinese five-spice powder and fresh ginger and then toss it with gluten-free soba or rice noodles, shredded chicken, scallions, soy sauce, and sesame oil for a quick Asian-inspired dinner.

- Enhance any pan gravy from a roast (beef, chicken, turkey, etc.) with a creamy sauce base (Creamy Mushroom Sauce makes a particularly good addition).

CREAMY CHICKEN SAUCE BASE

Makes 1¼ cups

1 tablespoon canola oil
1 cup coarsely chopped onion or shallots
2 cups low-sodium chicken broth
Salt and freshly ground black pepper

COOKS' NOTE:
Store sauce in tightly sealed container in refrigerator for 4 days or freezer for up to 2 months (do not add cream if freezing until sauce is reheated).

1. Heat the oil in a medium-sized, heavy saucepan over medium-high heat. Lightly sauté the onion until brown and caramelized, about 10 minutes.

2. Pour the broth into the saucepan. Increase the heat to high and bring to a boil. Reduce the heat to low and simmer, uncovered, for about 15 minutes. There should be about 10 ounces (1¼ cups) of liquid.

3. Pour the broth–onion mixture into blender and purée until smooth and creamy. Pour the puréed mixture back into the saucepan or a storage container and stir to combine. Season with the salt and freshly ground black pepper, to taste.

Variations

- Add about ½ teaspoon dried herbs, such as basil, dill, thyme, sage, tarragon, or oregano, while the broth is simmering.

- Add ¼ to ½ teaspoon of any spice, such as cumin, curry, chili powder, or Chinese five-spice powder, while the onions cook, if desired.

- Add 2 to 4 tablespoons light or heavy cream after the sauce is puréed.

- Add 1 to 2 tablespoons wine, sherry, or Port after the sauce is puréed.

Creamy Chicken Garlic Sauce Base

> 1 tablespoon canola oil
>
> 2 teaspoons minced garlic
>
> 1 cup coarsely chopped onion or shallots
>
> 2 cups low-sodium chicken broth
>
> Salt and freshly ground black pepper

1. Heat the oil in a medium-sized, heavy saucepan over medium-high heat. Lightly sauté garlic for 1 minute, until softened. Reduce the heat slightly; add onion and sauté until brown and caramelized, about 10 minutes.

2. Follow Steps 2–3 from the Creamy Chicken Sauce Base recipe on page 84.

CREAMY BEEF SAUCE BASE

Makes 1¼ cups

1 tablespoon canola oil

1 cup coarsely chopped onion or shallots

2 cups low-sodium beef broth

Salt and freshly ground black pepper

COOKS' NOTES:
Store the sauce in a tightly sealed container in the refrigerator for 4 days or the freezer for up to 2 months (do not add the cream until the sauce is reheated if you plan to freeze it).

1. Heat the oil in a medium-sized, heavy saucepan over medium-high heat. Lightly sauté the onion until brown and caramelized, about 10 minutes.

2. Pour the broth into the saucepan. Increase the heat to high and bring to a boil. Reduce the heat to low and simmer, uncovered, for about 15 minutes. There should be about 10 ounces (1¼ cups) of liquid.

3. Pour the broth–onion mixture into a blender and purée until smooth and creamy. Pour the puréed mixture back into the saucepan or a storage container and stir to combine. Season with the salt and freshly ground black pepper, to taste.

Variations

- Add about ½ teaspoon dried herbs (such as basil, oregano, or thyme) while the broth is simmering.

- Add ¼ to ½ teaspoon of any spice, such as cumin, curry, chili powder, or Chinese five-spice powder, while the onions cook, if desired.

- Add 2 to 4 tablespoons light or heavy cream after the sauce is puréed.

- Add 1 to 2 tablespoons wine, sherry, or Port after the sauce is puréed.

Creamy Beef Garlic Sauce Base

　　1 tablespoon canola oil

　　2 teaspoons minced garlic

　　1 cup coarsely chopped onion or shallots

　　2 cups low-sodium beef broth

　　Salt and freshly ground black pepper

1.　Heat the oil in a medium-sized, heavy saucepan over medium-high heat. Lightly sauté the garlic for 1 minute, until softened. Reduce the heat slightly; add the onion and sauté until brown and caramelized, about 10 minutes.

2.　Follow Steps 2–3 from the Creamy Beef Sauce Base recipe on page 86.

CREAMY MUSHROOM SAUCE BASE FOR GRAVY AND SOUP

Makes 2 cups

1 tablespoon canola oil

½ cup coarsely chopped onion or ¼ cup chopped shallots

8 ounces sliced mushrooms (domestic, shiitake, or crimini)

2 cups low-sodium chicken, beef, or vegetable broth

Salt and freshly ground black pepper

COOKS' NOTES:
Store the sauce in a tightly sealed container in the refrigerator for 4 days or in the freezer for up to 2 months. Do not add cream until the sauce is reheated if you plan to freeze it.

Take note: The mushrooms in this sauce will separate if frozen. If you intend to freeze it, add ¼ to ½ teaspoon guar gum (or xanthan gum) to the sauce while you purée it.

1. Heat the oil in a medium-sized, heavy saucepan over medium-high heat. Reduce the heat slightly; add the onion and sauté until lightly caramelized, 5 to 10 minutes. Set aside.

2. Add the mushrooms to the pan and sauté until they have softened and released their liquid. Return the onions to the pan and pour in the broth. Increase the heat to high and bring to a boil. Reduce the heat to medium and simmer, uncovered, about 20 minutes, until the vegetables are very soft. Reduce the sauce to about 2 cups of liquid, onion, and mushrooms combined.

3. Pour the broth–mushroom mixture into a blender and purée until smooth and creamy. Pour the puréed mixture back into the saucepan or a storage container and stir to combine. Season with the salt and pepper, to taste.

Variations

- Add about ½ teaspoon dried herbs, such as basil, thyme, sage, coriander, tarragon, or marjoram, while the broth is simmering.

- Add 2 to 4 tablespoons light or heavy cream after the sauce is puréed.

- Add 1 to 2 tablespoons wine, sherry, or Port after the sauce is puréed.

Creamy Mushroom Garlic Sauce Base

1 tablespoon canola oil

1 tablespoon minced garlic

½ cup coarsely chopped onion or ¼ cup chopped shallots

8 ounces sliced mushrooms (domestic, shiitake, or crimini)

2 cups low-sodium chicken, beef, or vegetable broth

Salt and freshly ground black pepper

1. Heat the oil in a medium-sized, heavy saucepan over medium-high heat. Lightly sauté the garlic for 1 minute, until softened. Reduce the heat slightly; add the onion and sauté until brown and caramelized, about 10 minutes.

2. Follow Steps 2–3 from the Creamy Mushroom Sauce Base recipe on page 88.

INTRODUCTION TO MAKING CREAMY SOUP BASES

You can use these rich, creamy bases to create a bountiful variety of fragrant soups. Add more broth, raw or cooked chicken or beef, vegetables, herbs, spices, potatoes, noodles, or rice, if you like. Top off your creation with a touch of wine, sherry, or cream for a bit of elegance. You can make the soup bases ahead of time and then store them in the freezer to pull out at the last minute, or make them when you need them. You will be able to create an incredible variety of flavorful soups at a moment's notice.

Ideas for using the creamy soup bases:

- Add the herb-infused Creamy Chicken Soup Base to more broth, bite-size chunks of potatoes, cooked chicken, and corn to create a rich, delicious chowder (see page 115).

- Use the Creamy Beef Soup Base to make a flavorful steak and potato chowder. Add the broth, marinated sliced steak, and bite-size chunks of potatoes. Top with shredded Gruyère cheese (see page 117).

- Mix the Creamy Chicken Soup Base with sake, fresh ginger, soy sauce, scallions, baby spinach, and cooked sliced chicken (marinated in hoisin sauce, a touch of sake, soy sauce, Chinese five-spice powder, garlic, and sesame oil) for an incredible Asian-inspired soup.

- Make the Creamy Chicken Soup Base with cumin and canned or fresh roasted chopped green chilies to create an enticing, Mexican-inspired soup made with shredded chicken, cooked white beans, corn, and chopped red and yellow peppers. Top it with shredded Monterey Jack cheese.

- Make the best beef pot pie you ever had by braising a chuck roast in red wine and/or broth until it's tender, cutting it into bite-size pieces, and combining it with the herb-infused Creamy Beef Sauce, cooked potatoes, mushrooms, peas, and carrots. Top it with a flaky pie crust (see page 219) or biscuits.

- Add chopped cooked chicken, potatoes, peas, and carrots to the herb-infused Creamy Chicken Sauce for a quick pot pie topped with a flaky pie crust (see page 219).

CREAMY CHICKEN SOUP BASE

Makes about 3 cups

> 1 tablespoon canola oil
> 1 cup coarsely chopped onion
> 1 cup coarsely chopped celery
> 1 cup coarsely chopped carrots
> 14–16 ounces low-sodium chicken broth (or homemade)
> Salt and freshly ground black pepper

1. Heat the oil in a large, heavy saucepan over medium-high heat. Add the onion, carrots, and celery and sauté until lightly caramelized. Add the broth. Increase the heat to high and bring to a boil. Cover the pan tightly. Reduce the heat to low and simmer for 15 to 20 minutes, until the vegetables are very soft.

2. Pour the broth/vegetable mixture into a blender and purée until smooth and creamy. Pour the puréed mixture back into the saucepan or a storage container and stir to combine. Season with the salt and freshly ground black pepper, to taste.

COOKS' NOTES:
Store the sauce in a tightly sealed container in the refrigerator for 4 days or in the freezer for up to 2 months.

Variations

- Add 2 to 3 tablespoons freshly chopped dill while broth is simmering, if desired.

- Add about 1 teaspoon (or to taste) of any dried herbs, such as basil, thyme, or oregano, while the broth is simmering.

- Add ¼ to ½ teaspoon of any spice, such as cumin, curry, chili powder, or Chinese five-spice powder, while the onions cook, if desired.

CREAMY BEEF SOUP BASE

Makes about 3 cups

1 tablespoon canola oil
1 cup coarsely chopped onion
1 cup coarsely chopped carrots
1 cup coarsely chopped celery
14–16 ounces low-sodium beef broth (or homemade)
Salt and freshly ground black pepper

1. Heat the oil in a large, heavy saucepan over medium-high heat. Add the onion, carrots, and celery and sauté until lightly caramelized. Add the broth. Increase the heat to high and bring to a boil. Cover the pan tightly. Reduce the heat to low and simmer for 15 to 20 minutes, until the vegetables are very soft.

2. Pour the broth/vegetable mixture into a blender and purée until smooth and creamy. Pour the puréed mixture back into the saucepan or a storage container and stir to combine. Season with the salt and freshly ground black pepper, to taste.

Variations

- Add about 1 teaspoon (or to taste) of any dried herbs, such as basil, thyme, or oregano, while the broth is simmering.

- Add ¼ to ½ teaspoon of any spice, such as cumin, curry, chili powder, or Chinese five-spice powder, while the onions cook, if desired.

OLD-FASHIONED SAUCEPAN CHICKEN GRAVY

Golden pan gravy made from the drippings of roast chicken is always delicious. But what to do when there aren't any drippings? Here's a quick and delectable gravy you can make in minutes to dress up simple baked, stuffed chicken breasts, complement store-bought rotisserie chicken, or spoon over hot open-faced chicken sandwiches. Add herbs, spices, and a touch of wine or cream, and you've turned everyday fare into something special. You can also combine it with pan drippings (if you've got them) to make a more robust version for roast chicken and mashed potatoes.

Makes 1¼–1½ cups

2 tablespoons unsalted butter

1½ teaspoons potato starch

1¼ cups Creamy Chicken Sauce Base or Creamy Chicken Garlic Sauce Base (see page 85)

¼ cup low-sodium chicken broth, optional, for a thinner gravy

¼ teaspoon dried, or 1 teaspoon fresh, herbs, optional

Salt and freshly ground black pepper

1. Melt the butter in a small, heavy saucepan over low heat. Mix the potato starch into the melted butter and cook slowly, stirring constantly, for 1 minute. Gradually stir in the Creamy Chicken Sauce Base (and extra broth and/or herbs, if using).

2. Increase the heat to medium and cook, stirring constantly, until the gravy is smooth and thick and reaches the boiling point. Allow the gravy to simmer for 1 to 2 minutes while stirring, and then season to taste with salt and pepper.

Variations

- Add 2 to 4 tablespoons light or heavy cream (substitute for additional broth in the ingredient list) after you simmer the gravy for 1 to 2 minutes, and then heat until hot.

- Add 1 to 2 tablespoons wine, sherry, or Port (substitute for additional broth in the ingredient list).

COOKS' NOTES:
Store the gravy in a tightly sealed container in the refrigerator for up to 4 days. The gravy can be frozen for up to 2 months only if the Creamy Chicken Sauce Base was not previously frozen (also, do not add cream until the gravy is reheated if you plan to freeze it).

OLD-FASHIONED SAUCEPAN BEEF GRAVY

Hungry for a hot roast beef sandwich? Looking for a perfect way to top off your holiday roast? Want to dress up meatloaf and mashed potatoes? This delectable gravy is comfort food at its best. You can add herbs, pan drippings, a touch of wine, or cream and create a mealtime favorite of your own.

Yields 1¼–1½ cups

2 tablespoons unsalted butter

1½ teaspoons potato starch

1¼ cups Creamy Beef Sauce Base or Creamy Beef Garlic Sauce Base (see recipes pages 86–87)

¼ cup low-sodium beef broth, optional, for a thinner gravy

¼ teaspoon dried, or 1 teaspoon fresh, herbs, optional

Salt and freshly ground black pepper

COOKS' NOTES:
Store the gravy in a tightly sealed container in the refrigerator for up to 4 days. The gravy can be frozen for up to 2 months only if the Creamy Beef Sauce Base was not previously frozen (also, do not add cream until the gravy is reheated if you plan to freeze it).

1. Melt the butter in a small, heavy saucepan over low heat. Mix the potato starch into the melted butter and cook slowly, stirring constantly, for 1 minute. Gradually stir in the Creamy Beef Sauce Base (and extra broth and/or herbs, if using).

2. Increase the heat to medium and cook, stirring constantly, until the gravy is smooth and thick and reaches the boiling point. Allow the gravy to simmer for 1 to 2 minutes while stirring, and then season to taste with salt and pepper.

Variations

- Add 2 to 4 tablespoons light or heavy cream (substitute for additional broth in the ingredient list) after you simmer the gravy for 1 to 2 minutes, and then heat until hot.

- Add 1 to 2 tablespoons red wine or cognac (substitute for additional broth in the ingredient list).

OLD-FASHIONED SAUCEPAN MUSHROOM GRAVY

This delicate gravy is infused with a rich mushroom taste. Use it to turn simple steamed vegetables into a dish that will have them coming back for seconds. Make homey casseroles or vegetable pot pies on cold winter nights. Spoon it over mashed potatoes and steak or roast chicken. It is versatile, delicious, and full of the powerhouse nutrients mushrooms are known for: Vitamin B, potassium, phosphorus, zinc, selenium, and copper.

Makes about 1⅓ cups

> 2 tablespoons unsalted butter
> 1½ teaspoons potato starch
> ½ cup milk
> 1 cup Creamy Mushroom Sauce Base (see page 88)
> ¼ teaspoon dried, or 1 teaspoon fresh, herbs, optional
> Salt and freshly ground black pepper

1. Melt the butter in a small, heavy saucepan over low heat. Mix the potato starch into the melted butter and cook slowly, stirring constantly for 1 minute. Gradually stir in the milk, Creamy Mushroom Sauce Base, and herbs, if using.

2. Increase the heat to medium and cook, stirring constantly, until the gravy is smooth and thick and reaches the boiling point. Allow the gravy to simmer for 1 to 2 minutes while stirring, and then season to taste with salt and pepper.

Variations

- Add 1 to 2 tablespoons red or white wine as a substitute for 1 or 2 tablespoons of the milk.

- Add 1 to 2 tablespoons light or heavy cream after you simmer the gravy for 1 to 2 minutes, and then heat until hot.

COOKS' NOTES:
Store the gravy in a tightly sealed container in the refrigerator for up to 4 days. The gravy can be frozen for up to 2 months only if the Creamy Mushroom Sauce Base was not previously frozen (also, do not add cream until the gravy is reheated if you plan to freeze it).

Take note: The mushrooms in this gravy will break down a bit when frozen. After you defrost the gravy, add ¼ teaspoon guar gum or xanthan gum and simmer in a small saucepan until thickened and hot.

ROUX

Roux is a kitchen classic. It is the foundation of a wide variety of sauces, soups, main dishes, hors d'oeuvres, and desserts, and you won't want to be without it in your repertoire. It's traditionally made with wheat flour, but potato starch is an acceptable substitute: it doesn't add a pronounced flavor, and it provides a nice, glossy finish to whatever you are making. Unlike wheat flour, potato starch does not need to be cooked for a long time in order to break down the gluten proteins and avoid a raw, pasty flavor.

Thin Sauce (also the base for Macaroni and Cheese, see page 176)

> 2 tablespoons butter
>
> 2 teaspoons potato starch
>
> 1 cup milk or broth

Thick Sauce

> 2 tablespoons butter
>
> 1 tablespoon plus 2 teaspoons potato starch
>
> 1 cup milk or broth

All-Purpose Sauce

> 2 tablespoons butter
>
> 4 teaspoons potato starch
>
> 1 cup milk or broth

COOKS' NOTES:
The starches in these rouxs can break down a bit when sauces made from them are reheated more than once or frozen. If this happens, you can add about ¼ teaspoon guar gum or xanthan gum (or a little more, if necessary) and then simmer the sauce in a saucepan until thickened and hot.

To make a white roux for a white sauce:

A gluten-free white roux is simply butter, potato starch, and milk or light stock. It is the starting point in many recipes for white sauces, soufflés, and classic cream soups.

1. Melt the butter in a medium-sized, heavy saucepan over low heat. Mix the potato starch into the melted butter and cook slowly, stirring constantly, for 1 minute (the roux will look foamy, not pastelike). Gradually stir in the milk or broth. Increase the heat to medium and cook, stirring constantly, until the white sauce is smooth and thick and reaches the boiling point. Reduce the heat. Add salt and pepper, to taste, if desired.

To make a dairy-free roux:

2. Use Smart Balance butter substitute and rice and/or soy milk in place of the butter and milk. Use higher-fat versions (64 percent or higher). The roux will not foam as described above; it will look more traditional and pastelike.

To make a brown roux for a brown sauce:

A brown roux is often made by stirring wheat flour into a mixture of butter, vegetables, bacon, or ham. Our gluten-free version can be made with butter alone, but you have to be sure not to cook it too long, or the starch will break down. It will take about 3 to 5 minutes for the butter and potato starch mixture to become a nutty brown color. This brown roux is an excellent base for Creole gumbos and stews. (Take note, dairy-intolerant readers: A Cajun roux is made with vegetable oil or lard and needs only 2 minutes to cook.)

1. Melt the butter in a medium-sized, heavy saucepan over medium-low heat. Mix the potato starch into the melted butter and cook slowly, stirring constantly, for 3 to 5 minutes, until the roux looks foamy and the butter mixture becomes a nutty brown color. Gradually stir in the milk or broth. Increase the heat to medium and cook, stirring constantly, until the brown sauce is smooth and thick and reaches the boiling point. Reduce the heat. Add salt and pepper, to taste, if desired.

CHEESE SAUCE

2 tablespoons unsalted butter

4 teaspoons potato starch

1 cup milk (whole is best)

2 cups (8 ounces) shredded cheese

Salt and freshly ground black pepper

1. Melt the butter in a medium-sized, heavy saucepan over low heat. Mix the potato starch into the melted butter and cook slowly, stirring constantly, for 1 minute. Gradually stir in the milk. Increase the heat to medium and cook, stirring constantly, until the white sauce is smooth and thick and has reached the boiling point. Reduce the heat; add the cheese, stirring until the cheese is melted. Season with the salt and pepper, to taste.

CHAPTER 6

Soups, Chowders, and Chilis —
Thinking Like a Hunter-Gatherer

SOUPS ARE AN EASY and nourishing way to get dinner on the table. A quick search around the kitchen for a few choice ingredients can lead to a bountiful variety of one-pot meals.

The idea of creating a soup around what you find in your larder isn't exactly new. Early man started many meals with a cooking pot, some bones, water, and whatever beans and vegetables could be foraged. Today, faced with busy days full of work, chores, and kids who need chauffeuring, we still hunt and gather. And just like those early cooks who had to do with whatever they could find, we have to be flexible and adaptable in order to get a meal on the table. We search for what we have on hand and enhance it with what looks fresh and delicious at the grocery store or farmers market. Here's where having a well-stocked pantry and a keen mind can relieve meal-time boredom and facilitate day-to-day cooking.

Black Bean Soup

Lentil Soup

Spanish Peasant Soup

Roasted Poblano–Asiago Soup

Roasted Winter Vegetable Soup

Creamy Mushroom Soup

Chicken, Corn, and Potato Chowder

Steak and Potato Chowder

Manhattan Clam Chowder

Dal (Curried Lentils)

Red Bean and Beef Chili

White Bean and Chicken Chili

THE SCIENCE OF CREATING SOUP

Bean Soups

Beans were so important to early diets that they were one of the first foods to be cultivated. Today, in our grocery store-oriented society, beans are the overlooked jewels of the vegetable world. They're inexpensive and are one of the best protein buys around. Combine them with whatever vegetables you happen to have on hand, or what looks most appetizing at the store, to create a sumptuous soup.

When we make our bean soups, we like to rely on more civilized flavor-enhancing techniques like sautéing or roasting garlic or vegetables to bring out their unique character. And although we often prefer to start with dry beans, we have come to rely on the ease and convenience of good-quality canned beans for a quick, nutritious, and delicious meal. But our modern-day bean soups use the same simple recipe as those of early man—a pot, beans, vegetables, and liquid and seasonings (you can even throw in a bone or two, if you want).

Here are a few simple steps:

1.   Sauté minced garlic and diced vegetables for 10 minutes in a stockpot until softened.*

2.   Add cooked or canned beans, liquid, and seasonings (including dry herbs).

3.   Simmer until tender and adjust the seasonings, to taste.

4.   Garnish with fresh herbs, scallions, grated cheese, and/or sprouts before serving.

Creamy Soups

We love the luxurious richness of a cream soup, but often find it too filling. Fortunately, it's possible to create flavorful creamy soups with less saturated fat by puréeing caramelized vegetables with stock and then adding just a touch of cream before serving (sometimes we don't even bother with the cream). When we're pressed for time during the week, we reach for one of our ready-made soup bases (see recipes in Chapter 5) and build a soup with whatever else we can find that appeals to our appetite. The steps are basically the same, but you will be able to start with Step 3 if you have a soup base on hand.

1.   Sauté 3 cups chopped vegetables (usually onions, carrots, and celery) for about 15 minutes, until softened (and sometimes caramelized, depending on the recipe).*

2.   Add 2 cups of stock or broth and cook the vegetables until they are very soft. Purée until smooth in a blender.

3.   Add more stock (per your recipe), seasonings (including dried herbs), and additional vegetables. Simmer until tender and adjust the seasonings, to taste.

4.   Add meat, poultry, or fish and fresh herbs and cook per your recipe.

*Some recipes call for a quick sauté of bacon. The cooked meat is removed and the vegetables are sautéed in the remaining fat. The crisp bacon pieces are then sprinkled over the finished dish.

5. Add cooked noodles or rice, if indicated, and garnish with fresh herbs, scallions, and/or grated cheese before serving.

Other Soups

The basic steps for most of the other soups you might be inclined to create use some combination of the steps we advocate for bean or creamy soups. We usually start with a quick sauté of vegetables (usually onions, celery, and carrots) and add stock or broth; more vegetables; seasonings; and meat, poultry (on or off the bone), or fish and simmer until tender. (Cooked meat, poultry, or fish can also be added after the vegetables are soft to make a really quick soup.) Fresh herbs are added at the very end to enhance the flavor.

THE ART OF CREATING SOUP

We've included many favorite soup recipes in this chapter, and we think you'll be able to find at least a few to add to your own repertoire. But we also encourage you to use the recipes as a starting point. Mix things up by throwing in some diced pancetta. Use different vegetables in the sauté. Change the herbs and spices. The Italian White Bean Soup you made last week can be flavored with fiery chipotle chilies and spicy sausage for this week's Mexican Black Bean Soup. Soup, chowder, and chili all lend themselves to infinite possibilities, but the components stay basically the same:

- Stock, broth, milk, or cream, and sometimes water
- Diced vegetables and aromatics (onions, carrots, celery, leeks, garlic, or shallots) sautéed in butter or oil
- Seasonings like spices and fresh or dried herbs
- Beans
- Meat, poultry, or fish
- Additional vegetables and starches (potatoes, rice, or noodles)
- Acids, such as vinegars or lemon or lime juice
- Other flavorings, such as tamari soy sauce, fish sauce, or hot sauce

So try a little hunting and gathering for your next meal, and enjoy this time-honored way of preparing food with family and friends.

MEASURING BEANS
One 15.5-ounce can of beans equals about 1½ cups of cooked beans. One cup of dried beans yields 3 cups cooked. One pound of dried beans yields 6 cups cooked.

BEAN POT BASE RECIPE
A favorite weeknight recipe in our homes is the Bean Pot. We choose a cuisine and then pick beans, herbs, spices, and meats to go along. Here is our basic recipe, with a few favorite variations at the end. The idea is to adjust the recipe to suit your particular taste (more beans, less spice, and so on).

Step 1: The Flavorings
> 1 tablespoon olive oil
>
> ½ cup chopped pancetta or smoked bacon, optional (depending on recipe)
>
> 1 tablespoon minced garlic
>
> 1–2 cups chopped onion
>
> ½–1 cup chopped green or red pepper, optional (depending on recipe)

1. Heat the olive oil in a large, heavy (5- to 6-quart) stockpot over medium-high heat. Reduce the heat to medium-low and sauté the pancetta or smoked bacon until softened. Remove the pancetta or smoked bacon from the stockpot and set aside in a medium-sized bowl. Add the garlic and onion and sauté for 5 minutes. Increase the heat to medium, add the green pepper, if using, and sauté for 5 minutes more. Set aside bowl (with pancetta or bacon if using).

Step 2: The Meat
> 1 teaspoon olive oil
>
> Meat options to total about 1¼ pounds:
>
> Chicken; turkey; tender cuts of pork, beef, or lamb cut into bite-size pieces; or ground chicken, turkey, beef, pork or lamb
>
> Sausage (kielbasa, andouille, chorizo, Italian, or French garlic, which could be made of turkey, chicken, pork, or soy) cut into bite-size pieces
>
> Smoked ham, diced

2. Add the olive oil to the stockpot and increase the heat to high (omit the oil if there is enough fat left over from the smoked bacon). Brown the meat or poultry on all sides. Remove from the stockpot and set aside in the medium-sized bowl (with flavorings and the smoked bacon/pancetta, if using). Add the sausage, if using, to the stockpot

and brown quickly on all sides. Add the smoked diced ham, if using, to the stockpot and quickly brown on all sides.

Step 3 Additions: The Beans, Broth, Seasonings, and Veggies

3–4 cups (about 2 cans) cooked chickpeas or red, white, or black beans

14–16 ounces (about 1 can) low-sodium broth

Seasonings (basil, thyme, oregano, cumin, chili, curry, and so on), to taste—see Seasonings Suggestions sidebar on this page

Salt and freshly ground black pepper

Vegetable Options in Place of or in Addition to Meat Options
(vegetable options to total about 2 cups (or 1 pound of greens):

½–1 pound chopped spinach or kale

½–1 pound butternut squash or other winter squash, cut into bite-size pieces

1–2 cups zucchini or other summer squash, cut into ½-inch-thick bite-size pieces

1–2 cups green or other beans

1–2 cups sweet or Yukon gold potatoes

3.   Add the broth, browned meat/poultry/soy, browned sausage, smoked ham, bacon or pancetta (if using), and all flavorings to the stockpot. Stir well to release the bits of browned meat from the bottom of the stockpot. Add the seasonings and vegetables and bring to a boil. Reduce the heat to very low and cover; simmer for 15 minutes, stirring occasionally. Add the beans and continue to simmer for another 30 to 45 minutes, with the cover partially off for a stewlike bean pot, or the cover closed for a soupier bean pot.

SEASONING SUGGESTIONS

French
¼ cup chopped fresh parsley
1 large bay leaf
1 teaspoon thyme leaves
¼ teaspoon allspice
⅛ teaspoon ground cloves

Cajun
¼ cup chopped fresh parsley
1 large bay leaf
½ teaspoon chili powder
½ teaspoon dried thyme
½ teaspoon dried basil
⅛–¼ teaspoon cayenne, or crushed red, pepper
⅛ teaspoon ground cloves

Indian
2 teaspoons minced peeled fresh ginger
1–2 teaspoons curry powder
1 teaspoon ground coriander
1 teaspoon ground turmeric

BLACK BEAN SOUP

Black bean soup is a year-round favorite. Ours is enhanced with sautéed vegetables, spices, and fresh herbs to make a rich, comforting soup that will leave you wondering why you don't make it more often. Serve it with brown rice, a touch of shredded cheese, and a big, fresh salad for a delicious and easy weeknight meal.

Serves 4 (recipe can be doubled)

2 tablespoons olive oil

1 cup chopped onion

2 teaspoons minced garlic

1 cup chopped green pepper

½ cup diced celery

1 tablespoon granulated sugar

2 cups cooked or canned black beans

2 cups low-sodium vegetable or chicken broth

1 bay leaf

1 tablespoon red wine vinegar

1 teaspoon soy sauce

1 teaspoon ground cumin

1 teaspoon freshly ground black pepper

½ teaspoon dry mustard

½ teaspoon ground coriander

1 ripe tomato, chopped, including juice

¼ cup chopped fresh cilantro

1. Heat the olive oil in a large, heavy (5- to 6-quart) saucepan over medium-high heat. Add the onion and garlic and sauté for 5 minutes. Add the green pepper and celery and sauté for 5 minutes more over medium heat.

2. Increase the heat to high and add the sugar. Stir continuously for 2 minutes.

COOKS' NOTES:
This soup can be made ahead of time and stored in the refrigerator for up to 3 days in a tightly sealed container. The leftovers can be stored in the refrigerator for up to 3 days and the freezer for up to 4 weeks in a tightly sealed container. Re-warm over medium-high heat.

3. Add the black beans, broth, bay leaf, vinegar, soy sauce, cumin, black pepper, dry mustard, coriander, and tomato. Bring to a boil. Reduce the heat, cover, and simmer for 20 minutes. Add the cilantro and adjust seasonings. Remove the bay leaf.

LENTIL SOUP

Lentil soup is a savory, neutralizing meal in a bowl. Not only are lentils one of the best vegetable sources of iron, they are also rich in magnesium, dietary fiber, and folic acid. They also have more protein than any vegetable except soybeans.

We like lentils because they are adaptable and versatile; their earthy flavor can be enhanced with herbs, spices, and any number of vegetables. Here is our own classic recipe for lentil soup, one that never fails to charm us and those around our table. But you can use it as the foundation to create your own more exotic version, with spinach, sausage, or any other flavors (for example, paprika with dashes of cinnamon, allspice, and cayenne).

4–6 servings (recipe can be doubled)

2 tablespoons olive oil

2 teaspoons minced garlic

1 cup chopped onion

½ cup chopped green pepper

½ cup chopped red pepper

½ cup minced celery

½ cup diced carrots

1 tablespoon granulated sugar

7 cups low-sodium chicken or vegetable broth

3 cups dried lentils, rinsed

2 teaspoons salt

1½ cups diced fresh, or 1 (14.5-ounce) can diced, tomatoes

2 tablespoons dry red wine

2 tablespoons lemon juice

1 teaspoon dried basil

1 teaspoon dried oregano

2 bay leaves

1 teaspoon freshly ground black pepper

¼ cup minced fresh parsley

Salt and freshly ground black pepper

1. Heat the olive oil in a large, heavy (5- to 6-quart) saucepan over medium-high heat. Add the garlic and onion and sauté for 5 minutes. Add the green and red pepper, celery, and carrots. Reduce the heat to medium and sauté for 5 more minutes.

2. Increase the heat to high and add the sugar. Stir continuously for 2 minutes. Transfer the cooked aromatics and vegetables to a bowl and set aside.

3. In same saucepan, add the broth, lentils, and salt and bring to a boil. Reduce the heat and simmer, covered, for 1 hour.

4. Uncover and add the cooked aromatics and vegetables, tomatoes, wine, lemon juice, basil, oregano, bay leaves, and pepper. Bring to a boil and then continue to simmer, covered, over low heat for 30 minutes. Remove the bay leaves, stir in the fresh parsley, and season with additional salt and pepper, to taste. Serve hot.

COOKS' NOTES:
This soup can be made ahead of time and stored in the refrigerator for up to 3 days in a tightly sealed container. The leftovers can be stored in the refrigerator for up to 3 days and the freezer for up to 4 weeks in a tightly sealed container. Rewarm over medium-high heat.

SPANISH PEASANT SOUP

Our colorful Spanish Peasant Soup is a beautiful blend of garbanzo beans and fresh vegetables accented with paprika, turmeric, basil, cinnamon, and cayenne. It can be prepared in less than 45 minutes, start to finish. Just one large bowlful will supply your body with three servings of vegetables and one large serving of beans. What more could you ask for? It is a nutritional powerhouse in an Impressionist landscape.

4–6 servings (recipe can be doubled)

2 tablespoons olive oil

2 cups chopped onion

2 cups peeled diced (into 1-inch pieces) sweet potato

½ cup diced celery

1 teaspoon minced garlic

3 cups low-sodium vegetable or chicken broth

1 teaspoon paprika

1 teaspoon ground turmeric

1 teaspoon dried basil

1 bay leaf

Dash ground cinnamon

Dash cayenne pepper

1½ cups diced fresh, or 1 (14.5-ounce) can diced, tomatoes

1 cup diced yellow pepper

1½ cups cooked chickpeas

1 teaspoon salt

½ teaspoon freshly ground black pepper

1. Heat the olive oil in a large, heavy (5- to 6-quart) saucepan over medium-high heat. Add the onion, sweet potato, celery, and garlic, and sauté for 10 minutes. Add the broth, paprika, turmeric, basil, bay leaf, cinnamon, and cayenne pepper.

COOKS' NOTES:

This soup can be made ahead of time and stored in the refrigerator for up to 3 days in a tightly sealed container. The leftovers can be stored in the refrigerator for up to 3 days in a tightly sealed container. Rewarm over medium-high heat.

2. Reduce the heat and simmer, covered, for 15 minutes. Add the tomatoes, yellow pepper, and chickpeas. Cover and simmer another 15 minutes, until vegetables are tender.

3. Remove the bay leaf. Season with the salt and pepper and serve hot.

Variation

•   Carrots or butternut squash can be substituted for the sweet potatoes.

ROASTED POBLANO–ASIAGO SOUP

Several years ago, we had the pleasure of dining at Steven Pyle's Restaurant in Dallas. The food and atmosphere were wonderful. Our favorite item that night was a Roasted Poblano–Asiago Soup. The next week, we tried to recreate the dish and we think we came pretty close. Either way, the soup is smooth and very satisfying; it's perfect on a hot summer night with a glass of wine.

Makes 4 servings (recipe can be doubled)

6 medium poblano chilies
4 medium tomatillos, paper-like husks removed
1 tablespoon unsalted butter
1 tablespoon olive oil
1½ cups chopped sweet onions
1 teaspoon minced garlic
3 cups low-sodium chicken broth
1 tablespoon chopped fresh cilantro
1 tablespoon chopped fresh basil
1 tablespoon chopped fresh mint
1 tablespoon chicken demi-glace*
¼ cup (or more) heavy cream
¼ cup shredded aged Asiago or Monterey Jack cheese
Salt and freshly ground black pepper

COOKS' NOTES:
This soup can be made ahead of time and stored in the refrigerator for up to 3 days in a tightly sealed container. The leftovers can be stored in the refrigerator for up to 3 days in a tightly sealed container. Rewarm over medium-high heat.

1. Char the poblano chilies over a gas flame or under a broiler until blackened on all sides. Enclose in a paper bag and let stand for 10 minutes to steam. Peel, seed, and chop the chilies.

2. Preheat the oven to 400°F. Place the rack in the bottom third of the oven. Roast the tomatillos on a small baking sheet (lined with foil for easy cleanup) for 10 minutes, or until lightly browned.

*We recommend More than Gourmet brand.

3. Heat the butter and olive oil in a medium-sized, heavy (3-quart) saucepan over medium-high heat. Add the onion and garlic and sauté until the onion is tender, about 5 minutes. Add the chilies and tomatillos and sauté for 1 minute. Add the broth and bring to a boil. Cover the pan. Reduce the heat to medium-low and simmer for 10 minutes, or until chilies are very tender.

4. Mix in the cilantro, basil, mint, and demi-glace. Working in batches, purée the soup in a food processor or blender. Return the soup to the pot and mix in the heavy cream and cheese. Season with the salt and pepper, to taste.

5. If the soup is too thick or spicy, add more cream, 1 tablespoon at a time. Serve hot.

ROASTED WINTER VEGETABLE SOUP

We enjoy eating rich, creamy vegetable soups in the cold weather. We love them for a delicious, hot lunch and even more so for a colorful, nutritious dinner. Our Roasted Winter Vegetable Soup is packed with health-giving vegetables: butternut squash is high in beta carotene, vitamin E, and potassium; parsnips help detoxify the body; leeks contain healing compounds that are antibacterial and antiviral; turnips are chock full of cancer-fighting compounds; and carrots contain high levels of carotenoids that help enhance the immune system and boost the body's ability to fight cancer and heart disease. Make up a pot of this soup as a treat for both your taste buds and your body.

Serves 6 (recipe can be doubled)

2 tablespoons olive oil

2 tablespoons maple syrup

1 tablespoon cider vinegar

1 teaspoon minced garlic

1 teaspoon coarse salt

1 teaspoon freshly ground black pepper

Pinch cayenne pepper

1 small butternut squash (about 2 pounds), peeled, seeded and cut into 1-inch cubes

3 leeks, white and light green parts only, cleaned, cut in half lengthwise and then into 2-inch lengths (see Cooks' Notes)

1 large parsnip, peeled and cut into 1-inch rounds (about 1 cup)

1 small yellow turnip, peeled and cut into 1-inch cubes (about 1 cup)

1 large carrot, peeled and cut into 1-inch rounds (about ½ cup)

5 cups low-sodium vegetable or chicken broth

2 small bay leaves (or 1 large)

½ teaspoon dried thyme leaves

1 teaspoon chopped fresh, or ½ teaspoon dried, rosemary

¼ cup heavy cream, optional

Salt and freshly ground black pepper

¼ cup grated Parmigiano-Reggiano or Gruyère cheese, for garnish

1. Preheat the oven to 425°F. Place the rack in the bottom third of the oven. Line a large baking sheet with foil and grease with oil or cooking spray.

2. In a large mixing bowl, combine the oil, maple syrup, cider vinegar, garlic, salt, pepper, and cayenne. Add the prepared vegetables and toss until coated in the mixture. Spread the vegetables in a single layer on the prepared baking sheet.

3. Place the baking sheet in the oven and roast, tossing occasionally, until the vegetables are tender and caramelized at the edges, about 30 to 40 minutes (if the vegetables are cold, add another 15 minutes).

4. Remove the baking sheet from the oven and transfer the vegetables to a large, heavy (5- to 6-quart) saucepan. Pour the broth into the pan and add the bay leaves, thyme leaves, and rosemary. Bring to a boil. Reduce the heat and simmer for 10 minutes. Remove and discard the bay leaves.

5. Transfer the soup to a food processor or blender and, working in batches, purée until thick and smooth. Add additional broth to thin the soup if desired. Return the soup to the saucepan. Add the heavy cream and season with the salt and pepper, to taste. Serve hot with the grated cheese.

COOKS' NOTES:
This soup can be made ahead of time and stored in the refrigerator for up to 3 days in a tightly sealed container. The leftovers can be stored in the refrigerator for up to 3 days in a tightly sealed container. Rewarm over medium-high heat.

To wash the leeks thoroughly, first cut off their tops and then cut them in half lengthwise before washing out the grit and sand.

CREAMY MUSHROOM SOUP

You can make this fabulous creamy mushroom soup in less than 30 minutes if you have our Creamy Mushroom Sauce Base on hand. It's so rich and flavorful that you'll never miss the half-and-half or heavy cream called for in other mushroom soup recipes. Serve it as an elegant first course, a nutritious lunch, or as part of a simple supper with a spinach salad on the side.

Serves 4–6 (recipe can be doubled)

1 tablespoon butter or canola oil

1 pound sliced mushrooms (domestic, shiitake, or crimini)

2 cups Creamy Mushroom Sauce Base (see page 88)

2 cups low-sodium chicken broth

2 tablespoons sherry or Madeira wine, optional

½ teaspoon dried thyme or 1½ teaspoons finely chopped fresh thyme

Salt and freshly ground black pepper

COOKS' NOTES:
This soup can be made ahead of time and stored in the refrigerator for up to 3 days in a tightly sealed container. The leftovers can be stored in the refrigerator for up to 3 days in a tightly sealed container. Rewarm over medium-high heat.

1. Heat the butter or oil in a large, heavy (5- to 6-quart) saucepan over medium heat. Add the mushrooms to the pan and sauté until they have softened and released their liquid.

2. Pour the Creamy Mushroom Sauce Base, broth, sherry (if using), and thyme into the saucepan; stir to combine. Cover and simmer for 10 minutes. Season with the salt and pepper, to taste. Serve hot.

CHICKEN, CORN, AND POTATO CHOWDER

When the weather gets cold, there's nothing better than sitting in front of the fire and eating a creamy chowder. A clear liquid soup won't do for these evenings. We want a thick soup brimming with potatoes, vegetables, and some bite-size chunks of meat. An old family favorite is our Chicken, Corn, and Potato Chowder. It's a thick, rich soup that's hearty enough to be a meal and so delicious that people will ask for more. It's also a great soup for children because there are no vegetables—except the corn, which most kids love—to pick out; all those tasty and healthy veggies are hidden in the Creamy Chicken Soup Base. Use a high-quality flash-frozen brand of corn; it's simply impossible to get good, fresh corn in the winter. We like to round out this meal with a big salad and hot homemade biscuits.

Serves 8

> ¼ pound bacon, diced
>
> 3 cups Creamy Chicken Soup Base (see page 91)
>
> 3 cups low-sodium chicken broth
>
> 2 tablespoons fresh dill
>
> 3 cups russet potatoes, skinned and cut into ½-inch cubes
>
> 2 cups fresh or defrosted frozen yellow corn kernels
>
> 3–4 cups cooked chicken cut into ½-inch cubes (about 1½–1¾ pounds uncooked chicken)*
>
> ½ cup light cream (or an additional cup low-sodium chicken broth)
>
> Salt and freshly ground black pepper

1. Cook the bacon over low heat in a large, heavy (5- to 8-quart) saucepan until crisp. Remove the bacon pieces and set aside in a small bowl. Drain all but 1 tablespoon of the fat from the saucepan.

*Here's a quick and easy method to cook the chicken: Place the raw cubed chicken in a large skillet. Turn the heat to medium, cover, and cook, stirring occasionally, until chicken is cooked through, about 10 minutes. Drain the liquid from the skillet and add the chicken to the soup.

COOKS' NOTES:
This chowder can be made ahead of time and stored in the refrigerator for up to 3 days in a tightly sealed container. The leftovers can be stored in the refrigerator for up to 3 days in a tightly sealed container. Rewarm over medium-high heat.

2. Combine the Creamy Chicken Soup Base, chicken broth, and dill in a large saucepan. Add the potatoes and corn and bring to a boil; reduce the heat, and simmer for 12 to 15 minutes, until the potatoes are just tender.

3. When the potatoes are tender, add the chicken and light cream (if using) to the broth mixture. Season with the salt and pepper, to taste. Cook for 3 minutes more until re-warmed. Ladle the chowder into bowls and sprinkle it with the bacon. Serve hot.

Variation

- To create a vegetarian version of this chowder, first prepare a Creamy Vegetable Soup Base using vegetable broth. Add the additional 3 cups vegetable broth and a soy-based meat substitute for the chicken. Substitute sweet potatoes for the russet potatoes.

STEAK AND POTATO CHOWDER

Steak and Potato Chowder is a kids-of-all-ages favorite. It combines sliced steak and potatoes in a rich, flavorful soup. The secret ingredient—our Creamy Beef Soup Base—lends to the hearty richness without even a hint of cream. We like to top it off with a bit of bacon and Gruyère cheese just before we set the bowls on the table. It takes only a bit of planning to marinate the steak ahead of time, but the requests for more will make you feel your time was well spent.

Serves 8

1¾ pounds boneless sirloin steak, sliced very thin (should have at least 1½ pounds after trimming)

½ cup chopped fresh flat-leaf parsley

2 tablespoons balsamic vinegar

1 tablespoon minced garlic

½ teaspoon dried thyme or 2 teaspoons fresh

⅓ pound bacon, diced

3 cups Creamy Beef Soup Base (see page 92)

3 cups low-sodium beef broth

1 tablespoon Worcestershire sauce

4 cups russet potatoes, skinned and cut into ½-inch cubes

Salt and freshly ground black pepper

½ cup shredded Gruyère cheese

1. Combine the sliced steak, parsley, vinegar, garlic, and thyme in a medium-sized bowl and mix well. Cover with plastic wrap and refrigerate overnight, or for at least 6 hours.

2. Cook the bacon over low heat in a large, heavy (6- to 8-quart) saucepan until crisp. Remove the bacon pieces and set aside in a small bowl. Drain all but 1 tablespoon of the fat from the saucepan.

3. Combine the Creamy Beef Soup Base, beef broth, and Worcestershire sauce. Add the potatoes, cover the saucepan and bring to a boil; reduce the heat and simmer for 12 to 15 minutes, until the potatoes are just tender.

COOKS' NOTES:
This chowder can be made ahead of time and stored in the refrigerator for up to 3 days in a tightly sealed container. The leftovers can be stored in the refrigerator for up to 3 days in a tightly sealed container. Rewarm over medium-high heat.

4. When the potatoes are tender, add the steak to the broth mixture and simmer 2 to 3 minutes more, until the steak is cooked. Add the salt and pepper, to taste. Ladle the chowder into bowls and sprinkle with the bacon and Gruyère cheese.

MANHATTAN CLAM CHOWDER

This soup is perfect for a quick midweek meal because it's so easy to make and satisfying to eat. If you've got clam juice, canned clams, and canned tomatoes in your pantry, as well as a few fresh vegetables and a touch of bacon, it's a snap to prepare. Although we love the idea of making it with sweet, fresh clams, the convenience of using canned is worthwhile. In only 30 minutes, you'll be able to sit down to a fragrant bowl of freshly made clam chowder. We like to serve it with a loaf of warm, crusty bread.

Serves 4 (recipe can be doubled)

2 slices bacon, diced

1 tablespoon unsalted butter

1 cup diced onions

1 cup diced celery

1 cup diced carrots

½ cup diced green pepper

1 (14.5-ounce) can diced tomatoes

2 cups bottled clam juice

1½ cups peeled diced potatoes

½ teaspoon dried thyme

13 ounces chopped canned clams, with juice

2 tablespoons chopped fresh parsley

Salt and freshly ground black pepper

1. Sauté the bacon in a large, heavy (5- to 6-quart) saucepan over medium heat until the fat is rendered and the bacon is soft and slightly browned on the edges.

2. Increase the heat to medium-high and add the butter. When the butter has melted, add the onions and sauté over medium heat for 5 minutes. Add the celery, carrots, and green pepper and sauté another 5 minutes, or until the onions are translucent.

COOKS' NOTES:
This chowder can be made ahead of time and stored in the refrigerator for up to 3 days in a tightly sealed container. The leftovers can be stored in the refrigerator for up to 3 days in a tightly sealed container. Rewarm over medium-high heat.

3. Add the tomatoes, clam juice, potatoes, and thyme. Bring to a boil; cover the pot and reduce the heat, simmering for 15 minutes.

4. Stir in the clams (and any juice), parsley, salt, and pepper and simmer uncovered for 5 minutes. Adjust the seasonings and serve hot with crusty bread.

DAL (CURRIED LENTILS)

Dal is a classic Indian dish that is simple to prepare. Packed with nutrition, it's a staple in most Indian households and is served at many meals. Our version is filled with herbs, spices, and vegetables that combine to make a rich, delicious dish you'll want to make over and over. We like it for an easy lunch with rice, or as part of a dinner with other vegetables and grilled fish or chicken.

Serves 4 (recipe can be doubled)

- 1 tablespoon olive oil
- 1 cup minced onion
- 2 teaspoons minced garlic
- 1 tablespoon curry powder
- 1 teaspoon fresh grated ginger
- 1 fresh medium-sized jalapeño pepper, seeded and minced
- 4 cups low-sodium vegetable broth
- 1½ cups diced fresh, or 1 (14.5-ounce) can diced, tomatoes, including juice
- 1 cup dried lentils, washed
- 1 medium-sized sweet potato, peeled and diced
- 1 teaspoon salt
- ¼ cup finely chopped fresh cilantro, for garnish
- Salt and freshly ground black pepper

1. Heat the olive oil in a large, heavy (5-quart) saucepan over medium-high heat. Add the onion, garlic, curry powder, ginger, and jalapeño pepper and sauté for about 4 minutes.

2. Add the broth, tomatoes, lentils, sweet potato, and salt and bring to a boil. Reduce the heat to medium; cover loosely and simmer until the lentils are tender, about 30 minutes.

3. Just before serving, add the cilantro and season with the salt and pepper, to taste. Serve warm.

COOKS' NOTES:
Lentils can be made ahead of time and stored in the refrigerator for up to 3 days in a tightly sealed container. The leftovers can be stored in the refrigerator for up to 3 days and the freezer for up to 4 weeks in a tightly sealed container. Rewarm over medium-high heat.

RED BEAN AND BEEF CHILI

Everyone has a favorite classic red bean and beef chili, and this is ours. It's not complicated to make, and it's very flexible as far as the ingredients are concerned. You can replace the meat with ground buffalo, turkey, or a soy substitute, and you can add a smoky flavor by throwing in some diced chipotle peppers. Hearty, flavorful, and satisfying, this is a chili you can serve at backyard campfires, weeknight dinners, or tailgate parties. It'll never fail you.

Serves 8 (recipe can be doubled)

2 tablespoons canola oil

2 cups chopped onions

1 cup chopped green pepper

1 tablespoon minced garlic

2 pounds ground beef (chuck)

2 (28-ounce) cans diced tomato, including liquid

1 (6-ounce) can tomato paste

2 tablespoons chili powder

1 tablespoon ground cumin

1 tablespoon dried basil

1 tablespoon dried oregano

1–2 tablespoons dark molasses

2 teaspoons salt

1 teaspoon freshly ground black pepper

3–3½ cups cooked red kidney beans (about two 15.5-ounce cans, drained and rinsed)

Grated Monterey Jack cheese and/or sour cream, for garnish

1. Heat the oil in a large, heavy (5- to 8-quart) saucepan over medium-high heat. Add the onion, green pepper, and garlic; cook until tender, about 7 minutes. Add the ground chuck and cook, stirring often, until well browned. Drain out most of the fat.

COOKS' NOTES:
This chili can be made ahead of time and stored in the refrigerator for up to 3 days in a tightly sealed container. The leftovers can be stored in the refrigerator for up to 3 days and the freezer for up to 4 weeks in a tightly sealed container. Rewarm over medium-high heat.

2. Reduce the heat to medium and stir in the diced tomato, tomato paste, chili powder, cumin, basil, oregano, molasses, salt, and pepper. Reduce the heat to low, cover and simmer over low heat for 30 minutes. Stir in the beans, cover, and simmer for another 30 minutes. Serve hot with the grated Monterey Jack cheese and/or sour cream.

WHITE BEAN AND CHICKEN CHILI

Leave those images of red beans and ground round behind and try our delicious White Bean and Chicken Chili. We let tomatillos and green chili peppers take the spotlight. This is a very special chili you'll find yourself craving again and again. Like all chili, it can be made ahead of time. We like to serve it with warm homemade corn muffins.

Serves 4 (recipe can be doubled or tripled)

4 medium tomatillos, paperlike husks removed

2 tablespoons olive oil, divided

1 cup chopped onion

1 tablespoon minced garlic

1½ pounds boneless, skinless chicken, cut into 1-inch chunks (dark meat gives a richer flavor)

1 teaspoon ground cumin

1 teaspoon dried oregano

1 (14-ounce) can low-sodium chicken broth

3 cups cooked white cannelloni beans (about two 15.5-ounce cans, drained and rinsed)

1 fresh jalapeño chili pepper, seeded and diced

1 cup whole green chili peppers (about 4), charred and chopped (if using canned, drain liquid)

2 tablespoons chopped fresh cilantro

1½ teaspoons sea salt

Freshly ground black pepper

1. Preheat the oven to 400°F. Place the rack in the bottom third of the oven. Line a baking sheet with foil, and roast the tomatillos on a baking sheet (lined with foil for easy cleanup) for 10 minutes, or until lightly browned. Allow to cool. When the tomatillos are cool, purée or mash them. Set aside in a small bowl.

2. Heat 1 tablespoon of olive oil in a large, heavy (5- to 6-quart) saucepan. Sauté the onions and garlic over medium heat until soft. Remove from the pan and set aside with the tomatillos.

COOKS' NOTES:
This chili can be made ahead of time and stored in the refrigerator for up to 3 days in a tightly sealed container. The leftovers can be stored in the refrigerator for up to 3 days and the freezer for up to 4 weeks in a tightly sealed container. Rewarm over medium-high heat.

3. Heat the remaining oil in the same saucepan. Add the chicken, increase the heat to medium-high, and sauté over medium-high heat until the sides are lightly browned. Add the cumin, oregano, onions, and garlic and stir for 1 minute.

4. Add the chicken broth, white beans, jalapeño pepper, green chili peppers, and roasted tomatillos. Bring to a boil and reduce the heat to low. Simmer, partially covered, for 1 hour. The chili should have the consistency of a thick stew.

5. Stir in the salt and cilantro; season with the black pepper, to taste. Serve hot.

CHAPTER 7

Vegetables and Side Dishes

VEGETABLES PLAY A BIG ROLE in neutralizing your body. They are alkalizing and help balance the acidity inherent in most of the meat, poultry, fish, and grains that are part of our daily meals. We give them a lot of space on our dinner plates. Fortunately, the essential nature of vegetables means they lend themselves to a wide array of cooking methods and seasonings. They come in every color of the rainbow and offer a variety of textures, flavors, and nutrients. We enjoy cooking them in showstopping ways that delight the palate and the eyes. Oven-roasted cauliflower and Brussels sprouts turn heads, butternut squash gratin brings even little kids back for seconds, and summer's fresh-off-the-farm grilled corn could become a meal in itself. Whether they're quick and simple or multistage masterpieces, make sure the vegetables you serve have a focal point on your table.

THE SCIENCE OF COOKING VEGETABLES

There are really only a few important things to know about cooking vegetables: buy the freshest, most flavorful vegetables you can find, eats lots of different colors, and don't overcook them. The longer a vegetable cooks, the more nutrients it will lose and the less flavorful it will be to eat. Many people, including some of our vegetarian friends, get into a rut and cook the same vegetables the same way several days a week. But a few simple cooking methods will give you a treasure trove of variety, especially if you use an interesting combination of seasonings.

Sturdier vegetables, such as potatoes, sweet potatoes, yams,

Roasted Vegetables

  Asparagus

  Broccoli

  Brussels Sprouts

  Carrots

  Cauliflower

  Fennel

  Kale

  Okra

  Potatoes

  Red, Yellow, and Orange Peppers

  Zucchini

Our Favorite Mixed Roasted Vegetables

Roasted Root Vegetables

Oven-Fried Sweet Potatoes

Spicy Roasted Ratatouille Spread

Grilled Vegetables

Grilled Asparagus with Feta Cheese

Asian-Style Grilled Vegetable Platter

winter squash, carrots, and other root vegetables, are the mainstays of purées, mashes, gratins, and soups. But for these firm, dense vegetables, roasting enhances their true flavors like no other method of cooking.

Medium-firm vegetables, such as broccoli; cauliflower; eggplant; green, red, yellow, and orange peppers; zucchini and yellow squash; fennel; corn; celery; and onions, are all excellent roasted, sautéed, or stir fried. Most can be easily grilled and all can be used in soups.

The flavors of *delicate vegetables*, such as sugar snap peas, green beans, wax beans, okra, asparagus, kale, spinach, and other greens are enhanced by simpler preparations like steaming and sautéing. We also encourage you to roast snap peas, okra, or asparagus because this method uniquely highlights their inherent sweetness and flavor as they caramelize.

THE ART OF COOKING VEGETABLES

The art of cooking vegetables is really about seasonal freshness and your flexibility in deciding what to choose. Today's supermarkets are stocked with produce from all over the world, but the best-tasting and most nutritious vegetables are the ones that have the most vibrant colors; that have been grown close by; and that look fresh, crisp, and firm. Often we need a certain vegetable for a certain recipe, but we usually buy what's fresh and featured for the week. Buy only the fresh vegetables you will

FLAVORFUL VEGETABLES

Try to load up your plate with vegetables dishes enhanced with spices and herbs. Herbs and spices are packed with nutrients, antioxidants, and disease-preventing phytochemicals. Use flavored oils (e.g., olive, walnut, sesame), vinegars (e.g., balsamic, raspberry, red wine) and sauces (e.g., soy sauce, fish sauce, hot sauce) to balance and highlight each dish. Mustards; lemon; lime and orange zest or juice; honey; maple syrup; and cheese can also be used to smooth and round out flavors.

Grilled Corn on the Cob

Mashed Potatoes

Creamy Corn Pudding

Green Bean Casserole

Spinach and Goat Cheese Pie

Butternut Squash Gratin

Ratatouille

Sautéed Shredded Zucchini and Yellow Squash

Green Beans with Shiitake Mushrooms

Sautéed Baby Spinach with Garlic

Kale with Puttanesca Sauce

Roasted Pear and Arugula Salad

Tomato, Mozzarella, and Grilled Red Onion Salad

Green Salads

> Baby Greens with Balsamic Vinaigrette

> Baby Greens with Warmed Goat Cheese, Toasted Walnuts, and Walnut Oil Vinaigrette

Bean Salads

> White Beans with Tomato and Red Onion

> Black Beans with Corn and Tomato

> Three Bean Salad

Thyme-Scented Green Olives

use within several days, because their vitamin and mineral content decreases over time. And wash everything before you eat it!

We supplement fresh, seasonal vegetables with frozen and canned vegetables. Frozen vegetables are often less expensive than fresh and can provide seasonal freshness in months when the vegetable isn't in season. Sometimes, they're a better choice—particularly when the fresh versions look wilted and soft. Frozen vegetables are harvested at their peak, cleaned, given a quick bath in boiling water to set their color, and frozen very quickly. Nutrient loss is minimal, and the freezing halts any further degradation. In addition, since they are already prepped, frozen veggies save time and mess on a busy night. We also like to use them in soups and stews. However, do take note: When we buy frozen vegetables, we buy them in their *natural form with no other ingredients*, such as preservatives, salt, seasonings, or sauces.

Unlike frozen vegetables, some canned vegetables are not as nutritious as their fresh counterparts. We stay away from those, such as canned peas and corn. However, many other types are nutritious and delicious. We make many of these staples in our pantry—in particular, canned tomatoes, beans, and artichoke hearts.

Some of our seasonal favorites include:

- **Winter**: Brussels sprouts, cabbage, carrots, onions, parsnips, potatoes, squash, sweet potatoes, and turnips.
- **Spring**: Asparagus, kale, new potatoes, radish, rhubarb, spinach, Swiss chard, and spring greens like leaf lettuce and watercress.
- **Summer**: Broccoli, cauliflower, celery, corn-on-the-cob, cucumber, eggplant, fennel, green peas, leeks, romaine lettuce, okra, peppers, pole beans, snow peas, and tomatoes.
- **Autumn**: Artichokes, corn, pumpkin, and red cabbage.

Final words. There is a perception in this country that fresh vegetables are expensive. In fact, it's usually cheaper to buy in-season fresh, frozen, or canned vegetables than processed, packaged foods. The art is in being flexible. We shop according to what's on sale and buy what looks good. If our local markets are featuring fresh broccoli and cauliflower, that's what we'll eat. If a local supermarket is running a special on canned Muir Glen Fire-Roasted Tomatoes—one of our favorites— we'll stock up.

READY-MADE DIPS

A great way to make sure you get enough fresh vegetables in your daily diet is to take advantage of the abundant assortment of delicious, nutritious, and ready-made dips sold in grocery and specialty stores everywhere. We like to have a platter of colorful, ready-to-eat vegetables and containers of baba ghanoush, hummus, or guacamole on hand for snack attacks (although we find ranch dressing seems to be a kid-pleasing favorite as well).

ROASTED VEGETABLES

Roasting is our favorite way to prepare vegetables. Roasting gives vegetables a rich, sweet flavor because the natural sugars present in the food become caramelized. It's an easy way to prepare a lot of different vegetables all at one time so they can be used throughout the week in various meals. In addition, roasting elevates vegetables from the sidelines to center stage. Large platters of colorful, fresh vegetables make it easy to fill an entire side of your dinner plate, throw together a hot soup, or accent any salad. They can be tossed with whole grains to jazz up a pilaf or pasta dish, or added to a risotto.

Almost any vegetable, except most leafy greens (excluding kale), can be roasted. We recommend roasting vegetables with similar cook times together on a single baking sheet. Buy fresh, in-season vegetables to obtain the best flavor and maximum nutrient content.

Roasting sturdy vegetables. Wash, peel (if desired), and cut them to the desired size. Brush or toss them with olive oil, canola oil, or a flavored oil. Add salt, pepper, herbs, or spices, or leave them plain. Roast them in the bottom third of the oven on a heavy cooking sheet at 425°F for 20 minutes to 1 hour, until tender and caramelized. If you have a convection oven, use the Convection Roast setting with the rack placed in the middle of the oven, or roast multiple pans on alternating racks.

Roasting medium-firm vegetables. Wash and cut them to the desired size. Brush or toss them with olive oil, canola oil, or a flavored oil. Add salt, pepper, herbs, or spices, or leave them plain. Roast them in the bottom third of the oven on a heavy cooking sheet at 425°F for 10 to 30 minutes, until tender and caramelized. If you have a convection oven, use the Convection Roast setting with the rack placed in the middle of the oven, or roast multiple pans on alternating racks.

Roasting delicate vegetables. Wash and toss them with olive oil, canola oil, or a flavored oil. Add salt, pepper, herbs, or spices, or leave them plain. Roast them in the bottom third of the oven on a heavy cooking sheet at 425°F for 10 to 15 minutes, until tender and caramelized. If you have a convection oven, use the Convection Roast setting with the rack placed in the middle of the oven, or roast multiple pans on alternating racks.

Convection ovens. If using a convection oven, place the rack in the center of the oven and preheat to 425°F. The roasting time may be reduced. You can also roast multiple baking sheets of vegetables at the same time by spacing racks to every other notch. The roasting time may increase.

Serving ideas. Arrange a colorful assortment of roasted vegetables on a large platter; any combination can be prepared ahead, covered, and held at room temperature for up to 4 hours before serving. Plan for leftovers so you can use them throughout the week; store in tightly sealed containers for several days in the refrigerator.

Roasted Asparagus

1 pound fresh asparagus, with each piece having the same diameter

Extra virgin olive oil

Freshly ground sea salt and black pepper

1. Preheat the oven to 425°F. Place the rack in the bottom third of the oven.

2. Wash, trim, and dry the asparagus. Place the asparagus on a shallow baking sheet large enough for them to lie in a single layer. Drizzle the olive oil over the asparagus and gently shake the baking sheet to coat each one. Place the baking sheet in the lower third of the oven. Roast for about 8 minutes for thin asparagus, 10 minutes for medium-sized asparagus, and 12 minutes for thicker asparagus, until tender, lightly browned, and caramelized. Shake the baking sheet to turn the asparagus halfway through the cooking time. Season with the salt and pepper, to taste. Arrange on a platter with other vegetables.

Roasted Broccoli

2 pounds broccoli crowns, cut into 2-inch wide florets with stem attached

2 tablespoons olive oil

Freshly ground sea salt and black pepper

2 tablespoons fresh grated cheese, optional

1. Preheat the oven to 425°F. Place the rack in the bottom third of the oven. Line the baking sheet with foil (if desired, for easy cleanup) and grease with cooking spray.

2. In a medium-sized bowl, toss the broccoli florets with the olive oil. Spread the broccoli florets evenly on the baking sheet and roast them in the lower third of the oven, stirring occasionally for 20 to 25 minutes, until they are quite brown and tender. Sprinkle them with the cheese and return them to the oven for 2 to 3 minutes. Season with the salt and pepper and serve hot or at room temperature. Arrange on a platter with other vegetables.

Roasted Brussels Sprouts

1 pint (about 1 pound) Brussels sprouts

3 tablespoons olive oil

Freshly ground sea salt and black pepper

1. Preheat the oven to 425ºF. Place the rack in the bottom third of the oven. Line a baking sheet with foil (if desired, for easy cleanup) and grease it with cooking spray.

2. Cut the stems off the sprouts and remove any hard outer leaves. If the sprouts are large, cut them in half. In a medium-sized bowl, toss the sprouts with the olive oil. Spread the sprouts evenly on the baking sheet and roast them in the lower third of the oven, stirring occasionally for 20 to 30 minutes, until they are quite brown and tender. Season with the salt and pepper and serve hot or at room temperature. Arrange on a platter with other vegetables.

Roasted Carrots

2 cups baby carrots

Extra virgin olive oil

Freshly ground sea salt and black pepper

1. Preheat the oven to 425ºF. Place the rack in the bottom third of the oven.

2. Wash and dry the carrots. Place them on a shallow baking sheet. Drizzle the olive oil over the carrots and gently coat each one. Place the baking sheet in the lower third of the oven. Roast for about 15 to 20 minutes, until they are tender, lightly browned, and caramelized. Season with the salt and pepper, to taste. Arrange on a platter with other vegetables.

Roasted Cauliflower

1 large (2-pound) head cauliflower, cut into 2-inch wide florets

3 tablespoons olive oil

1 tablespoon curry powder, optional

Freshly ground sea salt and black pepper

1. Preheat the oven to 425ºF. Place the rack in the bottom third of the oven. Line a baking sheet with foil (if desired, for easy cleanup) and grease it with cooking spray.

2. In a medium-sized bowl, mix the olive oil and curry powder, if using, until smooth. Add the cauliflower florets and toss until evenly coated. Spread them evenly on the baking sheet and roast them in the lower third of the oven, stirring occasionally for 20 to 30 minutes, until they are golden and tender. Season with the salt and pepper and serve hot or at room temperature. Arrange on a platter with other vegetables.

Roasted Fennel

> 2 small fennel bulbs, trimmed and cut in half, or 1 large bulb, trimmed and cut into 1½-inch pieces
>
> 2 tablespoons olive oil, divided
>
> Freshly ground sea salt and black pepper

1. Preheat the oven to 425°F. Place the rack in the bottom third of the oven. Line a baking sheet with foil (if desired, for easy cleanup) and grease it with cooking spray.

2. Place the fennel on the baking sheet and drizzle the pieces with 1 tablespoon of the olive oil.

3. Roast the fennel for 10 minutes, and then turn the pieces over. Drizzle on the remaining olive oil and roast for another 10 minutes, or until it is slightly charred at the edges. Season with the salt and pepper and serve hot or at room temperature. Arrange on a platter with other vegetables.

Variation

*   Add a splash of balsamic vinegar or lemon juice during the last 5 minutes of roasting for added sweetness and taste. Serve with shaved Parmigiano-Reggiano cheese.

Roasted Kale

> 4 cups firmly packed kale, washed, trimmed, and dried
>
> 1 tablespoon olive oil
>
> 1 teaspoon coarse sea salt
>
> ½ teaspoon freshly ground black pepper
>
> 1 tablespoon toasted sesame seeds

1. Preheat the oven to 425°F. Place the rack in the bottom third of the oven. Line a baking sheet with foil (if desired, for easy cleanup) and grease it with cooking spray.

2. Peel off the tough stems by folding the kale leaves in half, like a book, and stripping the stems off. In a large bowl, toss the leaves with the olive oil. Spread the leaves evenly on the baking sheet and roast them in the lower third of the oven for 5 minutes. Turn the kale over. Roast the kale for another 5 minutes, until the leaves turn brown and become paper thin and brittle. Season with the salt and pepper and sprinkle with the sesame seeds. Serve hot or at room temperature. Arrange on a platter with other vegetables.

Roasted Okra

1 pound fresh small whole okra (less than 3 inches long)

1 tablespoon olive oil

½ teaspoon coarse sea salt

½ teaspoon freshly ground black pepper

1. Preheat the oven to 425ºF. Place the rack in the bottom third of the oven. Line a baking sheet with foil (if desired, for easy cleanup) and grease it with cooking spray.

2. In a medium-sized bowl, toss the okra with the olive oil, salt, and pepper. Roast for 5 minutes or until brown and tender. After 5 minutes have passed, turn the okra once and continue roasting for 5 more minutes. Serve hot or at room temperature. Arrange on a platter with other vegetables.

Roasted Potatoes

8 small red-skinned new potatoes, each cut in half (see Cooks' Note)

2 tablespoons olive oil

1 teaspoon coarse sea salt

½ teaspoon freshly ground black pepper

1 tablespoon chopped fresh rosemary, divided, optional

1. Preheat the oven to 425ºF. Place the rack in the bottom third of the oven. Grease a medium-sized roasting pan with cooking spray.

2. In a large bowl, mix the oil, salt, pepper and half the rosemary. Toss in the potatoes and coat well. Transfer the potatoes to the pan and roast them for about 30 minutes, stirring once, until they are caramelized and tender. Transfer the potatoes to a serving plate and sprinkle them with the remaining rosemary. Serve hot.

COOKS' NOTE:
You can use peeled and cut-up russet potatoes in place of red skinned potatoes.

Roasted Red, Yellow, and Orange Peppers

> 2 red bell peppers, each of the same approximate size
>
> 2 yellow bell peppers, each of the same approximate size
>
> 2 orange bell peppers, each of the same approximate size

1. Preheat the broiler. Place the rack on the second shelf of the oven. Line a large baking sheet with foil.

2. Cut each pepper in half length-wise and remove the seeds and fibers. Place the peppers, open side down, on the foil-lined baking sheet and place the baking sheet on the bottom rack in the oven.

3. Broil the peppers for 15 to 20 minutes, until they are blackened around the edges and slightly blackened on top. The peppers should be tender to the touch. Remove the baking sheet from the oven and fold the foil over the peppers to create a pocket; tightly crimp and seal the edges. Allow the peppers to stand at room temperature for 20 minutes. Open the foil pocket and peel the skins off the peppers. Arrange on a platter with other vegetables.

Roasted Zucchini

> 2 medium-sized zucchini
>
> Extra virgin olive oil
>
> Freshly ground sea salt and black pepper

1. Preheat the oven to 425°F. Place the rack in the bottom third of the oven.

2. Wash, trim, and dry the zucchini. Cut each zucchini in half lengthwise. Cut each half into 3 sections. Place the zucchini on a shallow baking sheet. Drizzle the olive oil over the zucchini sections and gently coat each one; lay them, cut side down, on the baking sheet. Place the baking sheet in the lower third of the oven. Roast for about 12 minutes, until they are tender, lightly browned, and caramelized. Season with the salt and pepper, to taste. Arrange on a platter with other vegetables.

OUR FAVORITE MIXED ROASTED VEGETABLES

This is our all-time favorite roasted vegetable dish. We cook and serve it for weeknight suppers, small dinner parties, and large crowds. We multiply the quantities in equal proportions based on how much we want to make at a particular time. The vegetables are delicious hot or at room temperature and are even good reheated.

This is the perfect vegetable dish for entertaining because it can be made the day before. We recommend a combination of at least four vegetables plus an onion. Good choices include sliced red and yellow peppers, sliced zucchini and yellow squash, baby carrots cut in half, halved Brussels sprouts, and asparagus cut into 2-inch pieces.

4 cups assorted vegetables, cut into approximately 1¼-inch chunks

1 cup peeled cubed sweet onion, peeled and cut into approximately 1¼-inch chunks

2 tablespoons olive oil

1 tablespoon maple syrup

2 teaspoons minced garlic, optional

½ teaspoon coarse salt

¼ teaspoon freshly ground black pepper, or to taste

⅛ teaspoon cayenne pepper, optional

1. Preheat the oven to 425ºF. Place the rack in the bottom third of the oven. Line a large, shallow baking sheet with foil and grease with oil or cooking spray (the baking sheet should be large enough so the vegetables can be very densely packed in a thick single layer).

2. In a large mixing bowl, combine the oil, maple syrup, garlic (if using), salt, black pepper and cayenne pepper (if using). Add the cut-up vegetables and onion and toss until coated in the mixture.

3. Spread the vegetables on the prepared baking sheet. Roast, tossing occasionally, until the vegetables are lightly browned and caramelized, about 25 minutes.

COOKS' NOTES:
If not serving immediately, cover vegetables tightly to keep them moist. Mix gently to combine with liquid that has settled on the bottom of the platter. Store vegetables in a tightly sealed container in the refrigerator for up to 4 days.

ROASTED ROOT VEGETABLES

Try this enticing combination of colorful root vegetables with roast chicken, pork tenderloin, or lamb chops. Seasoned with a savory blend of herbs and a touch of mustard, we slow-roast these winter farmers' market favorites to bring out their natural sweetness. This versatile dish is for mature audiences; don't deprive yourself just because your kids wouldn't touch it with a ten-foot pole.

Serves 6

> 2 tablespoons olive oil
>
> 1 tablespoon whole-grain mustard
>
> 1 tablespoon chopped fresh herbs, such as rosemary or dill
>
> ½ teaspoon coarse sea salt
>
> ½ teaspoon freshly ground black pepper
>
> 1 pound small turnips, peeled and cut into 1½-inch pieces
>
> 1 pound small beets, peeled and cut into 1½-inch pieces
>
> 1 pound baby carrots, peeled (or 1½-inch pieces cut carrots)
>
> 1 large red onion, peeled and cut into 8 wedges

1. Preheat the oven to 400°F. Place the rack in the bottom third of the oven. Line a large baking sheet with foil and grease with cooking spray.

2. In a large bowl, whisk together the olive oil, mustard, fresh herbs, salt, and pepper. Add the cut vegetables to the marinade and toss to coat them well.

3. Spread the vegetables on the baking sheet. Roast for 30 to 45 minutes, or until brown and tender. Turn once while roasting. Transfer to a serving platter and serve hot or at room temperature.

OVEN-FRIED SWEET POTATOES

Fiber-rich sweet potatoes have anti-inflammatory benefits because they contain high levels of the antioxidant beta-carotene. We add a spicy twist of chili powder that will stimulate both your taste buds and your endorphins, the body's feel-good chemical. Live a little and roast a batch today. Serve it with a garlic-flavored mayonnaise.

Serves 4

> 3 tablespoons extra virgin olive oil
>
> 3 large sweet potatoes, peeled and sliced like steak fries
>
> 1 teaspoon coarse sea salt
>
> ½ teaspoon freshly ground black pepper
>
> ¼ teaspoon chili powder

1. Preheat the oven to 425ºF. Line a baking sheet with foil. Place the rack in the bottom third of the oven. In a large mixing bowl, drizzle the oil over the potatoes and toss to coat. Add the salt, pepper, and chili powder and toss again.

2. Place the sweet potato slices in an even layer on the baking sheet. Keep space between them so they get crispy on all sides. Use 2 baking sheets if necessary.

3. Place the baking sheet into the oven for 10 minutes and then flip the slices over. Return the sheet to the oven for 10 more minutes. They should be soft on the inside and brown on the outside. Serve hot.

COOKS' NOTE:
In place of chili powder, you can also use 1 teaspoon ground cumin or 1 teaspoon curry powder.

SPICY ROASTED RATATOUILLE SPREAD

Our Spicy Roasted Ratatouille Spread serves as the basis for a variety of dishes: as a zesty spread for crackers; mixed with goat cheese for a quick and tasty pasta; served as a condiment alongside roasted meat, fish, or poultry; as a spread in a delicious sandwich; and even as a flavorful addition to a colorful salad topped with fresh, creamy cheese. You can make up a large batch to use as a party hors d'oeuvre, and then use the extra for a quick and easy weekday meal. It's a fresh, nutritious alternative to any store-bought, ready-made spread.

Yields 2–3 cups

¼ cup extra virgin olive oil

1 tablespoon minced garlic

½ tablespoon coarse sea salt

½ teaspoon black pepper

¼–½ teaspoon dried crushed red pepper

1 (1-pound) eggplant, peeled, cut into ¾-inch cubes

2 medium-sized red bell peppers, seeded, cut into ½-inch pieces

1 large red onion, peeled, cut into ¾-inch cubes

¼ cup sun-dried tomatoes packed in oil

1 tablespoon chopped fresh parsley

1 tablespoon chopped fresh basil

1. Preheat the oven to 425°F. Place the rack in the center of the oven. Grease a large baking sheet with cooking spray.

2. In a large bowl, whisk the oil with the garlic, salt, black pepper, and crushed red pepper.

3. Add the eggplant, bell peppers, and onion. Toss to coat. Spread the mixture on the baking sheet.

4. Roast the vegetables for 10 minutes and then turn. Continue to roast for another 10 to 15 minutes, or until the vegetables are tender and lightly browned. Cool for 10 minutes on the baking sheet.

5. Transfer the vegetables to the food processor. Add the sun-dried tomatoes, parsley, and basil. Pulse to process the vegetables until a coarse purée forms. Transfer the mixture to a bowl and adjust the seasonings to taste.

6. Allow the spread to stand at room temperature for 1 hour before serving. Serve with crispy crackers.

Roasted Meat, Fish, or Poultry with Spicy Roasted Ratatouille Purée

- Serve several tablespoons of warmed Spicy Roasted Ratatouille Spread as a purée alongside each serving of roasted meat, fish, or poultry.

Chicken, Turkey, Roast Beef, or Lamb Sandwiches with Spicy Roasted Ratatouille Spread

- Use 1 or 2 tablespoons of Spicy Roasted Ratatouille as a spread on chicken, turkey, roast beef, or lamb sandwiches.

Salad Greens with Spicy Roasted Ratatouille Spread and Fresh, Creamy Cheese

- Toss the salad greens with a balsamic vinaigrette (see page 160) and divide it onto salad plates. Place 1 or 2 tablespoons of Spicy Roasted Ratatouille Spread on top of the dressed greens and sprinkle them with a fresh, creamy cheese, such as goat or feta cheese.

Pasta with Spicy Roasted Ratatouille and Goat Cheese

Serves 4

> 4 cups dried fusilli or farfalle pasta
> 1½ cups Spicy Roasted Ratatouille Spread (see recipe on page 138)
> ½ cup low-sodium vegetable or chicken broth
> 4 ounces goat cheese
> ½ cup grated Parmesan cheese
> Salt and freshly ground black pepper

1. Cook the pasta in a large pot of boiling water until tender. Drain the pasta; do not rinse it with cold water. Return the pasta to the pot.

2. Place the saucepan containing the pasta over medium-low heat. Add the Spicy Roasted Ratatouille, broth, goat cheese, and Parmesan cheese and stir until well incorporated. Reduce the heat, cover the saucepan, and allow the pasta to cook for 1 minute more, until heated through. Add the salt and pepper, to taste. Serve immediately.

GRILLED VEGETABLES

Almost any vegetable can be grilled: whole potatoes wrapped in foil, unshucked corn, zucchini and yellow squash cut in half, slices of eggplant and onions, skewered baby Portobello mushrooms, and even whole green beans on a foil-lined grate. We usually grill vegetables over medium to medium-high direct heat.

Grilling sturdy vegetables. Wash, peel (if desired), and cut them to the desired size. Brush or toss them with olive oil, canola oil, or a flavored oil. Add salt, pepper, herbs, or spices, or leave them plain. Grill them directly on the grate or a grate covered with a foil at 425°F for 20 minutes to 1 hour, until tender. Turn every 10 minutes while cooking.

Grilling medium-firm vegetables. Wash and cut them to desired size. Brush or toss them with olive oil, canola oil, or a flavored oil. Add salt, pepper, herbs, or spices, or leave them plain. Grill them directly on the grate or in a grill basket at 425°F for 10 to 30 minutes, until tender and lightly brown. Turn every 5 minutes while cooking.

Grilling delicate vegetables. Wash and toss them with olive oil, canola oil, or a flavored oil. Add salt, pepper, herbs, or spices, or leave them plain. Grill them directly on the grate or in a grill basket at 425°F for 10 to 15 minutes, until tender and lightly brown. Turn every 2 to 3 minutes while cooking.

Serving ideas. Drizzle balsamic vinegar or your favorite vinaigrette over the grilled vegetables. Sprinkle them with chopped fresh herbs, such as basil, rosemary, thyme, or parsley, and season with coarse salt and freshly ground black pepper. Serve hot or at room temperature.

GRILLED ASPARAGUS WITH FETA CHEESE

This delectable dish is a perfect example of a simple recipe escalated to "Wow, you're a great cook" status. A ladies' favorite, we serve it as a hors d'oeuvre or as a side dish with grilled fish, poultry, or meat.

Serves 4–6

    2 pounds medium-sized asparagus, trimmed

    1 tablespoon extra virgin olive oil

    ½ teaspoon sea salt

    ½ teaspoon freshly ground black pepper

    ½ cup feta cheese, crumbled (you can use plain or flavored feta)

1. Preheat the grill to 425°F. Grease with olive oil.

2. Toss the asparagus with the oil, salt, and pepper. Place on the grill, perpendicular to the grates, in a single layer. Roast, turning every 3 minutes, until the asparagus is just tender when pierced with a fork, about 10 minutes.

3. Place the asparagus on a platter and sprinkle with the feta cheese. Serve hot or at room temperature.

ASIAN-STYLE GRILLED VEGETABLE PLATTER

Asian-inspired seasonings and colorful vegetables converge on the grill; serve this delicious platter alongside grilled meats, chicken, or fish. If you have a small grill, cook the vegetables first, transfer them to a platter, and cover them to keep them warm; then prepare the meat, poultry, or fish. Grilled vegetables can be held at room temperature for up to 4 hours.

Serves 6–8

Asian Marinade

2 tablespoons soy sauce

2 tablespoons rice wine vinegar

2 tablespoons sesame oil

2 tablespoons finely chopped fresh coriander

½ teaspoon freshly ground black pepper

Use any combination of vegetables from the list below:

2 Japanese eggplant, peeled below stem and cut length-wise from stem

2 medium-sized onions, peeled and cut in thin round slices

2 small zucchini (firm), washed and cut in half length-wise

2 small yellow squash (firm), washed and cut in half length-wise

3 Portobello mushrooms, washed

1 green pepper, cut in half length-wise and seeds removed

1 red pepper, cut in half length-wise and seeds removed

¼ cup olive oil

Salt and freshly ground black pepper

1. Combine the 5 marinade ingredients and mix well.

2. Pour ¼ cup of the marinade over the eggplant and let sit for 1 hour.

3. Spread the sliced onions horizontally on a sheet of foil. Drizzle them with olive oil and season with the salt and pepper. Seal the foil closed.

4. Drizzle the other vegetables lightly with olive oil and season with the salt and pepper.

5. Prepare the grill and coat the grates with olive oil. Grill the peppers, the packet of onions, and the eggplant at 425ºF for 20 minutes, turning every 5 minutes. Grill the zucchini, yellow squash, and mushrooms at 425ºF for 10 to 15 minutes, turning once, until fork-tender.

6. Slice the cooked mushrooms and peppers and toss lightly with the marinade. Cut the stems off the eggplants. Cut the zucchini, squash, and eggplants into smaller pieces. Arrange all vegetables on a platter and serve all vegetables warm or at room temperature.

GRILLED CORN ON THE COB

Dry heat and smoky flavors make grilled corn a perfect sweet vegetable companion to grilled beef. Sometimes we soak the corn in the husk for 20 minutes prior to cooking, but if it's "Jersey fresh," we just throw it on the top rack of the grill and cook away.

Serves 10

> 10 fresh corn cobs
> ½ cup (1 stick) butter
> Coarse sea salt and freshly ground black pepper

1. Preheat the grill to 400°F.

2. Pick ears of corn that are fresh, young, tender, and still in the husks. Remove all but the last 3 or 4 husks from each ear of corn. Place on the grill for about 4 minutes per side. Turn several times while grilling to expose all sides of the corn to heat. Cook for 12 to 16 minutes.

3. After cooking, remove the corn silks. Then, pull back the husks and tie them back with a strip of husk to make a handle. The corn should be firm, with a nice golden, roasted color.

4. Spread on the butter and season with the salt and pepper, to taste.

MASHED POTATOES

We make our "everyday" mashed potatoes without the heavy cream that dominates many restaurant versions by using low-fat milk. Adjust the butter amount to suit your taste and serve this homey comfort food with such classic fare as roast chicken, steak, or pork tenderloin.

Serves 4

> 2 pounds potatoes, peeled and cubed (about 1½ by 2-inch-wide cubes)*
>
> 2–4 tablespoons butter or margarine
>
> ½–¾ cup warm milk
>
> Salt and freshly ground black pepper

1. Place the potatoes in a heavy, large saucepan, cover with cold water, and bring to a boil over high heat.

2. Reduce the heat slightly and cook until the potatoes are tender, about 20 minutes. Drain the potatoes. Return the potatoes to the pot and mash until smooth.

3. Add the butter and milk and stir over low heat until the butter melts. Add more milk if the potatoes are too thick. Season with the salt and pepper to taste and serve hot.

COOKS' NOTES:
Can be made 2 hours ahead of time. Transfer to microwavable serving bowl and cover with plastic wrap. Let stand at room temperature. Before serving, add 2 tablespoons of milk or butter and stir; heat until hot in the microwave.

*Equivalent to about 4 large baking potatoes. Other options include Yukon Gold, Red Bliss, or white potatoes.

CREAMY CORN PUDDING

Creamy Corn Pudding is a cross between a cornbread and a pudding. It will hold its own in a supporting role to our pulled pork (see page 242), or you can serve it with your favorite barbecued meat. It can also costar with a spinach salad for a light vegetarian meal. We use frozen sweet baby corn kernels to ensure consistency in both taste and texture. Frozen corn kernels are also easier to use than cutting the corn off the cob, so prep time is a quick 10 minutes. And if there are any young aspiring chefs in the house, this corn pudding recipe is a great way to get their hands dirty because it's simple to prepare and serve. For extra flavor, add a ¼ cup of diced green chilies.

Serves 6–8

½ cup white or yellow corn meal

1 tablespoon granulated sugar

1 teaspoon baking soda

½ teaspoon sea salt

½ teaspoon dried thyme

1½ cups buttermilk*

½ heavy cream

4 large eggs

2 tablespoons unsalted butter, melted

3 cups defrosted, frozen white or yellow sweet baby corn kernels

1 tablespoon chopped fresh dill, optional

1. Preheat the oven to 350ºF. Place the rack in the center of the oven. Grease an 11- × 7-inch baking dish with cooking spray.

2. Whisk together the corn meal, sugar, baking soda, salt, and thyme in a large bowl.

3. Pulse the buttermilk, cream, eggs, and melted butter in a blender or food processor until smooth. Add the corn and dill and pulse a few more times (the mixture should be lumpy, with visible corn kernels).

4. Whisk the buttermilk mixture into the corn meal mixture. Pour into the prepared baking dish and bake for 30 to 35 minutes, until the edges are golden brown and the center remains slightly jiggly. Transfer to a rack to cool. Serve warm or at room temperature.

* You can use 6 tablespoons powdered buttermilk in 1½ cups water in place of the buttermilk.

GREEN BEAN CASSEROLE

Here is our very own version of that all-time holiday classic—the much-loved green bean casserole. Devoid of fat and gluten-laden canned soup, our version tucks the green beans into a nutrient-rich Mushroom Gravy made with our Creamy Mushroom Sauce Base. You can top the casserole with the ready-made onion-flavored crunch of Funyuns or invest a little more effort and make homemade onion rings (see Cooks' Note at left). As much as we try to avoid highly processed foods, putting Funyuns on top makes this a very kid-friendly dish.

Serves 6

> 1–1¼ cups Old-Fashioned Saucepan Mushroom Gravy (see page 95)
>
> 1 pound cooked green beans
>
> Salt and freshly ground black pepper
>
> ½ cup Funyuns, gently crushed

1. Preheat the oven to 350ºF. Place the rack in the center of the oven. Grease a 1½-quart casserole dish with cooking spray.

2. Combine the Mushroom Gravy, green beans, salt, and pepper in a medium-sized bowl. Spoon the mixture into casserole dish and top with the Funyuns. Bake at 350ºF for about 30 minutes, or until hot and bubbly. Serve immediately.

COOKS' NOTE:
To make onion rings, dip freshly sliced onion rings in a beaten egg, coat with plain rice flour, and then fry in hot oil until golden brown.

SPINACH AND GOAT CHEESE PIE

Our Spinach and Goat Cheese Pie is a dietician's delight. Packed with the super foods spinach and tofu, this dish makes for a perfect vegetarian lunch or supper. It is a favorite for potluck luncheons and a great alternative to brown bag sandwiches. Pack it for a ready-to-eat room temperature lunch at work or school.

Serves 4 as a main dish or 6 as a side dish

1 pound fresh spinach

2 bunches scallions

3 tablespoons butter

1 teaspoon minced garlic

½ teaspoon dried thyme

1 tablespoon chopped fresh basil

1 tablespoon chopped fresh parsley

Salt and freshly ground black pepper

1 cup silken tofu

5 ounces goat cheese

3 large eggs

1 cup milk

Ground nutmeg

¼ cup freshly grated Parmesan cheese

1. Preheat the oven to 375°F. Place the rack in the center of the oven. Grease a 9-inch pie pan with cooking spray.

2. Remove the stems from the spinach and cut the leaves into large pieces. Wash and spin dry.

3. Trim the roots and most of the greens off the scallions and thinly slice them.

4. Melt the butter in a large fry pan. Add the scallions, garlic, thyme, basil, and parsley, and cook over medium heat for 1 minute.

5. Gradually add the spinach by the handful. Let each batch of spinach soften and wilt before adding the next. Season with the salt and pepper and set aside.

6. In a food processor, purée the tofu. Add the goat cheese and blend until smooth. Then add the eggs and milk. Sprinkle on the nutmeg and season with more salt and pepper, to taste. Blend until well combined.

7. Mix the spinach mixture and custard together in a bowl and spoon into the prepared pan. Sprinkle with the Parmesan cheese. Bake at 375°F for 30 minutes, or until set and lightly browned. Allow to rest for 5 minutes before serving.

BUTTERNUT SQUASH GRATIN

We reduced the fat but not the flavor in this winter classic. Our savory gratin features roasted butternut squash, a sweet, nutty vegetable that's high in antioxidants but low in calories. This dish is a wonderful compliment to roasted meat and poultry. We also like to serve it alongside a white bean salad for a hearty vegetarian option. To save prep time, buy the peeled and precut fresh squash found in the chilled produce aisle.

Serves 6

2 tablespoons olive oil

1 tablespoon maple syrup

1 teaspoon minced fresh garlic

½ teaspoon coarse salt

½ teaspoon freshly ground black pepper

1 pinch cayenne pepper

4 cups butternut squash (about 2 pounds), peeled, seeded, and cut into 1-inch cubes

1 cup peeled and diced sweet onion

½ cup chicken broth

½ cup grated Parmigiano-Reggiano cheese

2 tablespoons heavy cream

1 tablespoon chopped fresh sage (or ½ teaspoon dried)

½ teaspoon dried thyme

Salt and freshly ground black pepper

1. Preheat the oven to 425°F. Place the rack in the bottom third of the oven. Line a large baking sheet with foil and grease with oil or cooking spray.

2. In a large mixing bowl, combine the oil, maple syrup, garlic, salt, pepper, and cayenne pepper. Add the squash and onions and toss until coated in the mixture.

3. Spread out the vegetables in a single layer on the prepared baking sheet. Roast, tossing occasionally, until the vegetables are lightly browned and caramelized, about 25 minutes.

4. While the vegetables are roasting, combine the broth, cheese, cream, sage, and thyme in a medium-sized mixing bowl. Set aside.

5. Remove the vegetables from the oven and toss with the broth mixture in the bowl. Transfer to a medium-sized casserole dish and bake at 400ºF for 20 minutes. Season with the salt and pepper, to taste. Serve hot.

RATATOUILLE

Decades ago, ratatouille was one of the first multivegetable recipes we ever made using fresh-picked eggplant, squash, tomatoes, and peppers from our own gardens. Back then, we simply layered slices of colored vegetables in a casserole dish with olive oil and Italian spices and baked it in the oven for an hour.

Our updated version has a greater depth of flavor. In fact, this time-honored dish is perfect for parties because if it's made in advance, it becomes even more flavorful the next day. Use leftovers to make a delicious goat cheese sandwich on rustic flat bread to accompany a Sunday-afternoon glass of red wine.

Serves 6

¼ cup olive oil

1 tablespoon minced garlic

1 cup chopped onion

1 small eggplant, peeled and cubed

1 tablespoon granulated sugar

1 green or orange bell pepper, cored, seeded, and cut into 1-inch squares

1 red pepper, cored, seeded, and cut into 1-inch squares

1 zucchini, cut into 1-inch cubes

1 yellow squash, cut into 1-inch cubes

6 plum tomatoes, diced, or 1½ cups diced canned plum tomatoes

1 tablespoon tomato paste

3 tablespoons dry red wine

1 teaspoon dried basil or ½ cup chopped fresh basil

1 teaspoon dried oregano

1 teaspoon dried marjoram

1 bay leaf

½ cup chopped fresh flat-leaf parsley

1 teaspoon salt

½ teaspoon freshly ground black pepper

1. Heat the oil in a large, heavy skillet over medium-high heat and add the garlic, onion, and eggplant. Sauté until the eggplant is soft and the onion is transparent, about 10 minutes.

2. Increase the heat to high and add the sugar. Stir constantly for 1 minute. Add the peppers, zucchini, and squash and cook for 2 minutes at medium-high heat.

3. Add the tomatoes, tomato paste, red wine, basil, oregano, marjoram, and bay leaf. Simmer, covered, for 20 minutes. Add the parsley, salt, and pepper. Stir well to combine and serve. Can be served hot, at room temperature, or cold.

COOKS' NOTE:
Ratatouille can be made up to 2 days in advance. Refrigerate until needed.

SHREDDED ZUCCHINI AND YELLOW SQUASH CAKES

By the end of the summer season, we're constantly looking for interesting ways to cook and serve the abundant quantities of fresh zucchini and summer squash that are piled high at farm stands everywhere. This recipe is a delicious change of pace because it dresses up an otherwise staid vegetable into fancy little cakes seasoned with garlic and basil.

Serves 4

1 tablespoon butter or margarine

2 teaspoons minced garlic

2 teaspoons dried, or 2 tablespoons minced fresh, basil

1½ cups thinly sliced onion

1½ cups packed shredded zucchini

1½ cups packed shredded yellow squash

Salt and freshly ground black pepper

COOKS' NOTES:
You can also serve the zucchini and squash mixture without pressing it into cakes. Simply reheat in a tightly covered skillet over medium-low heat or in the microwave, covered lightly with wax paper, until hot, and serve.

1. Melt the butter in a large skillet over medium heat. Stir in the garlic and basil, and then the onion. Sauté until the onions are tender, about 5 minutes. Add the zucchini and squash and sauté over medium-high heat until the liquid evaporates, another 6 to 7 minutes. Season with pepper and salt, to taste.

2. Press the mixture into four ½-cup ramekins or custard cups. At this point, the cakes can be reheated until hot in a microwave (see Step 3) or refrigerated up to 1 day for later use (see Step 4).

3. If using right away: Place the ramekins in the microwave and cover lightly with wax paper. Heat on high until warmed through, about 1 to 2 minutes. To serve, carefully turn each ramekin over onto individual dinner plates.

4. If refrigerated: Cover the ramekins tightly with plastic wrap and store in the refrigerator. When ready to use, remove the plastic wrap. Place the ramekins in the microwave and cover lightly with wax paper. Heat on high until warmed through, about 3 to 4 minutes. To serve, carefully turn each ramekin over onto individual dinner plates.

GREEN BEANS WITH SHIITAKE MUSHROOMS

Tired of the same old green bean dishes? Try our Green Beans with Shiitake Mushrooms. This fragrant dish is a snap to make and an exotic alternative to the popular green bean casserole featured on many holiday tables (see page 150). It goes well with roast beef or chicken, and makes an excellent accompaniment to grilled steak.

Serves 8

> 2 tablespoons butter, divided
>
> 8 ounces fresh shiitake mushrooms, sliced
>
> 2 medium shallots, chopped
>
> 1 teaspoon minced garlic
>
> 2 pounds slender green beans, trimmed
>
> ⅔ cup canned low-sodium chicken broth
>
> Salt and freshly ground black pepper
>
> 2 tablespoons fresh parsley

1. Melt 1 tablespoon of the butter in a large, heavy skillet over medium-high heat. Add the mushrooms and sauté until tender, about 5 minutes. Transfer to a bowl and set aside.

2. Melt the remaining butter in the same skillet. Add the shallots and garlic and sauté until tender, about 2 minutes.

3. Add the green beans and toss to coat with the butter. Pour the broth over the green beans. Cover and simmer until the liquid evaporates and the green beans are tender but crisp, about 10 minutes.

4. Stir in the shiitake mushrooms. Season to taste with the salt and pepper. Sprinkle with the parsley. Serve hot.

SAUTÉED BABY SPINACH WITH GARLIC

Most top-ten superfood lists contain spinach, a leafy green vegetable rich in vitamin A and C, protective phytochemicals, and neutralizing minerals, such as calcium, potassium and zinc. We developed this weeknight recipe as an example of a quick marriage between nutrition and flavor. Serve it with grilled, roasted, or sautéed meat and seafood, or tossed with brown rice and Parmesan cheese.

Serves 2–4

2 tablespoons extra virgin olive oil, divided

1 teaspoon minced garlic

1 tablespoon raw pine nuts

4 cups baby spinach leaves, washed, stemmed, and loosely packed

Salt and freshly ground black pepper

1. Heat 1 tablespoon of the olive oil in a heavy, medium-sized sauté pan over medium heat. Sauté the garlic and pine nuts for 60 seconds.

2. Add the spinach, salt, and pepper to the pan and cook for 90 seconds. Pour the liquid from the pan. Toss with the remaining olive oil. Serve hot.

KALE WITH PUTTANESCA SAUCE

We're not going to lie. Kale was not high on our list of most requested vegetables. But once we realized kale was one of the most neutralizing leafy green vegetables, we gave it another look—and boy, are we glad we did! Kale contains organosulfur phytonutrients that appear to lessen the occurrence of certain cancers, including breast and colon cancer. In addition, kale is an excellent source of vitamins A, C, and K and manganese, and it's also a very good source of fiber and calcium. We paired this nutritional powerhouse with a house-favorite pasta sauce to up the likability factor.

Serves 6 as a side dish

¼ cup extra virgin olive oil

2 teaspoons finely chopped garlic

1 (15-ounce) can fire-roasted crushed tomatoes

¼ cup white wine or low-sodium broth

½ cup Kalamata olives, halved and pitted

1½ tablespoons drained capers

1 teaspoon dried oregano

½ teaspoon dried crushed red pepper

1 pound kale, center ribs removed, leaves thinly sliced (about 8 cups)

2 tablespoons chopped fresh Italian parsley

Salt and freshly ground black pepper

2 tablespoons grated Parmesan cheese

2 tablespoons chopped pine nuts, toasted

1. Heat the oil in a large, heavy saucepan over medium heat. Add the garlic and sauté until fragrant, about 1 minute. Add the crushed tomatoes, white wine, olives, capers, oregano, and crushed red pepper. Cover and simmer the sauce over medium-low heat for 5 minutes.

2. Add the kale, cover, and continue to simmer for 10 minutes, or until the kale is tender. Stir in the parsley. Season with the salt and pepper, to taste. Garnish with the Parmesan cheese and pine nuts and serve warm as a side dish, or tossed with pasta.

ROASTED PEAR AND ARUGULA SALAD

Our sister who lives in Spain served a simple no-pear version of this gem several years ago for a Christmas party, and it's been one of our go-to salads ever since. We use it as a sophisticated start to a family dinner, or to charm a large crowd. The secret ingredient is walnut oil, a richly flavored specialty oil containing omega-3 essential fatty acids and vitamin E. In the summer, we substitute the roasted pears for fresh slices of avocado and serve it as a side salad with grilled meats.

Serves 4

2 Bartlett pears, cored and cut into eighths

2 teaspoons olive oil

4 cups arugula

¼ cup walnut oil

Coarse sea salt

Freshly ground black pepper

¼ cup shaved Parmesan cheese

¼ cup sliced almonds

COOKS' NOTE:
For richer flavor, toss the pears with balsamic vinegar and oil before roasting.

1. Preheat the oven to 450°F. Place the rack in the bottom third of the oven. Lightly grease a small baking sheet with cooking spray.

2. Toss the pear quarters in the olive oil. Roast at 450°F until slightly browned on both sides (5 minutes). *Cool slightly but use warm on the salad.*

3. Toss the arugula with the pears and walnut oil. Season with salt and pepper, to taste.

4. Place the salad on serving plates and sprinkle with the cheese and nuts.

TOMATO, MOZZARELLA, AND GRILLED RED ONION SALAD

This salad is great to serve at a barbecue in the summer, when luscious, ripe tomatoes are available at farm stands. Splurge on fresh artisan mozzarella cheese and top it off with high-quality olive oil and balsamic vinegar. The subtle flavors blend together to create a richly satisfying salad that is striking in its simplicity.

Serves 10

> 3 large red onions, cut into ½-inch thick slices
>
> 4 fresh tomatoes, sliced ¼-inch thick
>
> 20 slices fresh mozzarella cheese, ¼-inch thick
>
> 2 tablespoons chopped fresh basil
>
> ½ teaspoon coarse sea salt
>
> ½ teaspoon freshly ground black pepper
>
> 2 tablespoons extra virgin olive oil
>
> Balsamic vinegar, to taste

1. Preheat the grill to 425°F. Brush with olive oil.

2. Arrange the onion slices on the grill and roast for 5 minutes, or until the skins begin to char. Remove from the grill and set aside to cool.

3. Arrange the tomato, cheese, and onion slices on a serving platter. Sprinkle with the basil and season with the salt and pepper.

4. Drizzle with the olive oil and balsamic vinegar; serve immediately.

GREEN SALADS

Everyone should have a couple of fabulous mixed green salads in their repertoire, and these are ours. The dressings take only a few minutes to make, so you can have head-turning salads on the table in no time. Wash the baby greens, throw in some cheese, and use ready-made toasted nuts from the store if you want to skip a step. These salads are a staple in our homes. Try them and you'll see why.

Baby Greens with Balsamic Vinaigrette

Serves 4

> ½ cup walnuts or pecans
>
> 8 cups mixed baby greens
>
> 1 medium apple or pear, cut into bite-size chunks
>
> 4 ounces crumbled Gorgonzola, Roquefort, blue cheese or Montrachet (goat cheese)
>
> Balsamic Vinaigrette (recipe follows)

1. Preheat the oven to 350°F. Place the rack in the center of the oven.

2. Place the walnuts or pecans on a small baking sheet and bake at 350°F for 5 to 7 minutes, until lightly toasted. Set aside. (This can be done several days ahead; if you do, store the nuts in a tightly sealed container at room temperature until you use them.)

3. Toss the baby greens, fruit, and cheese with the Balsamic Vinaigrette. Arrange on salad plates. Sprinkle the top of each salad with the nuts.

Balsamic Vinaigrette

> ¼ cup extra virgin olive oil
>
> 3 tablespoons balsamic vinegar
>
> 1 tablespoon honey
>
> ¼ teaspoon salt
>
> ¼ teaspoon pepper

1. Combine all ingredients and shake to mix. Keep tightly covered and refrigerated. Allow to come to room temperature before using.

Baby Greens with Warmed Goat Cheese, Toasted Walnuts, and Walnut Oil Vinaigrette

Serves 4

> ½ cup walnuts
>
> 8 cups mixed baby greens
>
> 2 tablespoons toasted bread crumbs*
>
> 4 ounces goat cheese, sliced into 4 rounds
>
> Walnut Oil Vinaigrette (recipe follows)

1. Preheat the oven to 350ºF. Position the rack in the center of the oven.

2. Place the walnuts on a small baking sheet and bake for 5 to 7 minutes, until toasted. Set aside. (This can be done several days ahead; if you do, store the nuts in a tightly sealed container at room temperature until you use them.)

3. Grease a small baking sheet lightly with cooking spray. Carefully press the bread crumbs on to each round of goat cheese. Place the cheese rounds on a baking sheet and warm them in the oven for 3 minutes.

4. Toss the salad with the Walnut Oil Vinaigrette. Arrange on salad plates. Sprinkle the top of each salad with walnuts and place a warmed round of goat cheese on the side of each plate.

Walnut Oil Vinaigrette

> ½ cup walnut oil
>
> 3 tablespoons white wine vinegar or white balsamic vinegar
>
> ¼ teaspoon salt
>
> ¼ teaspoon black pepper

1. Combine all ingredients and shake to mix. Keep tightly covered and refrigerated. Allow to come to room temperature before using.

---

* An economical, easy to make gluten-free bread crumb recipe is available in *Gluten-Free Baking Classics, Second Edition*, by Annalise Roberts (Surrey Books, 2008). You can also simply grind up the ends of a loaf of gluten-free bread in a blender or food processor and then bake the crumbs in the oven at 325°F until lightly browned.

BEAN SALADS

We love bean salads. They are nutritious, inexpensive, and for whatever reason, men seem to gravitate to them—especially when they're served with barbecued meat. They are also versatile: the beans, vegetables, herbs, and spices can be varied to blend with any meal. We use a combination of fresh and high-quality convenience foods (such as frozen corn and green beans) to make our salads with less effort. The following recipes are three favorites, the ones we make all the time. Use them as a template for your own creations: change the ingredients, but not the proportions. Adaptable, simple, and a crowd pleaser—what more could anyone want from a side salad?

White Beans with Tomato and Red Onion

Serves 8 as a side dish

> 2 (15.5-ounce) cans cannelloni beans (about 3–3½ cups)
>
> 1½ cups firm ripe tomatoes, seeded and diced*
>
> ⅓ cup red onion, finely diced
>
> ⅓ cup extra virgin olive oil
>
> 2 teaspoons dried oregano or 2 tablespoons minced fresh oregano
>
> Sea salt and freshly ground black pepper

1. Rinse the beans with water and drain well. Blot with a paper towel to remove as much moisture as possible. Place the beans in a medium-sized bowl and add the tomato and onion. Toss with the olive oil and oregano.

2. Season with the salt and pepper, to taste. Serve at room temperature. Can be made up to 1 day ahead. Cover tightly and refrigerate. Allow to rise to room temperature before serving.

Variations

- Add crumbled feta or goat cheese.
- Substitute basil for the oregano.

---

* If good-quality tomatoes are not available, use cherry or grape tomatoes.

Black Beans with Corn and Tomato

Serves 4 as a side dish

> 1 (15.5 ounces) can black beans
>
> ¾ cup corn kernels (if frozen, thawed)
>
> 3 medium-sized plum tomatoes, seeded and cut into little pieces
>
> 4 medium-sized scallions, thinly sliced
>
> 2 tablespoons chopped fresh cilantro
>
> 3 tablespoons olive oil
>
> 1 tablespoon red wine vinegar
>
> 1 teaspoon ground cumin
>
> Sea salt and freshly ground black pepper, to taste

1. Rinse the beans with water and drain well. Blot with a paper towel to remove as much moisture as possible. Place the beans in a medium-sized bowl and add the corn, tomatoes, scallions, and cilantro. Toss with the olive oil, red wine vinegar, and cumin. Season with the salt and pepper, to taste. Serve at room temperature. Can be made up to 1 day ahead. Cover tightly and refrigerate. Allow to come to room temperature before serving.

Variation

- Omit 3 medium-sized plum tomatoes and substitute with 1 cup drained Muir Glen Organic Fire-Roasted Diced Tomatoes.

Three Bean Salad

Serves 8

12 ounces frozen whole green beans, thawed and drained

1 (15.5-ounce) can garbanzo beans, rinsed and drained

1 (15.5-ounce) can red kidney beans, rinsed and drained

¼ cup olive oil

2 tablespoons fresh lemon juice

2 tablespoons red wine vinegar

1 teaspoon minced garlic

¼ cup chopped fresh parsley

1 tablespoon chopped fresh herbs (such as dill, basil, or thyme)

1 teaspoon coarse salt

Freshly ground black pepper

1. Cut the green beans in half from the center, on an angle.

2. In a medium-sized mixing bowl, combine the cut green beans, garbanzo and red kidney beans, olive oil, lemon juice, red wine vinegar, garlic, parsley, and fresh herbs.

3. Season with the salt and pepper and chill for at least 2 hours.

4. Add more salt and pepper, if needed. Serve cold or at room temperature.

THYME-SCENTED GREEN OLIVES

This recipe reminds us why we love tapas bars. Even though many supermarkets now feature fresh olives, the zest of homemade marinated olives is worth the extra effort. Serve them with a favorite wine and enjoy the rich flavor. Prepare this dish several days in advance—it gets better with time.

> 7 ounces large green Spanish olives
>
> ¼ cup olive oil
>
> 2 cloves garlic, lightly crushed and peeled
>
> 1 tablespoon dried thyme
>
> 1 teaspoon lemon zest
>
> ¼ teaspoon freshly ground black pepper

1. Crush the olives lightly with the flat side of a broad knife.

2. Combine the olives with the olive oil, garlic, thyme, lemon rind, and pepper in a covered plastic or glass container. Cover tightly and shake to mix. Keep at room temperature for 24 hours and then refrigerate for at least 2 days. To serve, bring the olives to room temperature.

CHAPTER 8

Grains

Unlike most people in america, grains do not comprise
the bulk of our daily food. Oh, we eat them, but not as the
centerpiece of every meal. If we have pancakes for breakfast, we also serve lots of fresh fruit, yogurt, and maybe
some humanely raised bacon on the side. If we eat some
gluten-free pizza for lunch, a green salad and slices of fresh
fruit will fill the left side of the plate. If pasta is dinner, it
shares the stage with lots of vegetables and protein.

THE SCIENCE OF COOKING GRAINS

Grains are the seed-bearing fruit of grasses. We eat them
in two forms: whole and refined. Whole grains contain
the entire grain kernel (the germ, bran, endosperm, and
hull) and are more nutritious than refined grains, which
have been milled to remove the germ and bran. Grains
are high in carbohydrates and provide your body with energy, although whole grains also naturally contain varying
amounts of protein, fats, vitamins and minerals.

There is a great deal of controversy about eating grains.
Some leading grain-based food organizations believe we
should eat a lot of grains. On the other hand, some pro-
moters of low-carbohydrate diets frown on the consumption of all grains. Adding to the confusion are whole-grain
advocates (who include most cereal companies, dietitians,
and health professionals) who promote studies that suggest
whole-grain eaters have lowered risk of cancer, diabetes,
and heart disease. Of course, most people who eat whole
grains also usually eat more fruits and vegetables, so let the

buyer beware—researchers have yet to prove that it's the whole grains, and not the fruits and vegetables, that make the difference. However, research has proven that diets high in refined grains—even gluten-free refined grains—can cause chronic inflammation, which is the pathway to obesity and disease.

When we do cook with grains, we go gluten free. We try to use whole grains, like brown rice pasta, steel cut oats, brown rice, quinoa, and millet, whenever possible in a recipe. But some recipes just don't work with whole grains. A creamy risotto requires white arborio rice. Buckwheat pancakes need a mixture of both whole and refined grains for texture and taste. Gluten-free breads need starches to lighten the millet, oat and sorghum flours. So, we recommend experimenting and trying different gluten-free grains to find the ones that work for you and your family. And don't sacrifice taste for fiber. Get your fiber from vegetables, fruits and nuts, and not grains. Think of grains as a beloved food accessory—they make a meal more fun, but they aren't necessary.

THE ART OF COOKING GRAINS

Grain preparation is simple and usually involves two cooking techniques: boiling and simmering (see Chapter 4, page 72). Perhaps the only trick to cooking grains is to make sure the grains are fresh and not rancid. Whole grains go rancid within 3 to 6 months, so only buy what you need or store whole grains tightly sealed in the refrigerator or freezer. Rancid grains often have a nutty, oily smell and a bitter taste.

When preparing whole grains, it is important to thoroughly rinse them before cooking to remove dirt. We offer the following easy steps:

1. Pour the grains into a heavy pot (with a tight-fitting lid), cover with cold water, and swish the pot in a circular motion. Then, drain the grains into a colander and rinse with cold water.

2. Return the grains to the pot. Add the proper amount of water for cooking and a pinch of sea salt for flavor. Bring the contents of the pot to a boil, lower the heat to a simmer, and continue to cook, covered, for the specified time, depending on the type of grain. Whole-grain cook times vary anywhere from 15 minutes to 45 minutes. Cut oats and white rice cook in 15 minutes. Quinoa cooks in 20 minutes. Brown rice cooks in 45 minutes.

3. When the grains are done, remove the pot from the heat. Stir, cover, and let rest for 2 minutes.

Gluten-free pasta is tricky. Many brands are mushy, sticky, or bitter tasting. It's important to find a brand you like and luckily, this task is getting easier and easier as the market for gluten-free foods expands. A tried and true choice for the price is Tinkyada Brown Rice Pasta. Schar Pasta, a brand from Italy, has the best-tasting corn pastas currently on the market, but the brand is often difficult to find and more expensive. Whichever brand becomes your favorite, we offer the following steps to assure success each time:

1. Use a large pot and 1 gallon of water per pound of pasta. The more water you use, the less gummy the pasta will be.

2. Bring the water to a hard boil. If you want to add salt, add it *after* it boils at a rate of 2 teaspoons per pound.

3. Add the pasta in batches, and stir between batches to keep the pasta from sticking.

4. Cook the pasta *al dente*—not too soft, and not too hard. Fresh pasta cooks very fast (2 to 6 minutes) and dried pasta requires 8 to 20 minutes, depending on its size and shape. You need to begin to taste for doneness halfway through the recommended cooking time on the box or package. Use a long-handled spoon or fork to remove a strand from the boiling water.

5. When the pasta is done, drain it in a large colander, giving it a few quick shakes. Do not rinse.

6. Have the sauce ready unless you are making a room-temperature pasta dish. Toss the cooked pasta with the sauce and serve hot. Otherwise, you should toss the pasta in a bowl with some butter or olive oil if you cannot immediately add the sauce.

Risotto is a true comfort food that's ready in less than 30 minutes. And if you start with a high-quality short-grained rice, like arborio, vialone, or carnaroli, it can take a little abuse. We offer the following steps to assure perfect risotto—or almost perfect—every time:

1. Do not rinse the rice before cooking it. The starch that coats each grain is essential for making a creamy risotto.

2. Use a heavy, flat-bottomed pot that won't burn.

3. In a separate saucepan, keep the broth at a simmer. (Sometimes when rushed, we warm it in the microwave.)

4. After 15 minutes, begin to check the rice to see if it is *al dente*. It should be tender and creamy with a slight chewiness to it, not mushy or sticky.

5. When the risotto is done, cover the pot, remove it from the heat, and let it rest for 2 minutes.

CHICKEN NOODLE GRATIN

The soothing essence of potato gratin and the creamy simplicity of chicken and noodles are artfully combined in this dish. Gruyère cheese tops noodles and chicken tossed in a rich, flavorful sauce made with our Creamy Chicken Garlic Sauce Base. It's perfect for a weeknight meal but good enough to serve anytime. This dish will become a favorite.

Serves 6

1½ pounds skinless boneless chicken breasts, cut into large bite-size pieces

2 teaspoons minced garlic

¼ cup Newman's Own Olive Oil and Vinegar Dressing*

1 tablespoon olive oil

1¼ cups Creamy Chicken Garlic Sauce Base (see page 93)

¼ cup light cream

4 cups fusilli or penne pasta

Salt and freshly ground black pepper

8 ounces Gruyère cheese, shredded

Ground nutmeg, to taste

1. Place the chicken pieces and garlic in a medium-sized bowl and coat with the dressing. Cover and refrigerate overnight, or for at least 2 hours (overnight is best).

2. Preheat the oven to 375°F. Place the rack in the center of the oven. Grease a large gratin dish or a 9- × 13-inch baking dish with cooking spray. Combine the Creamy Chicken Garlic Sauce Base and cream and set aside.

3. Heat the olive oil in a large, heavy skillet over high heat (you can also use a large, heavy (5-quart) saucepan in order to avoid a lot of cleanup). Add the cut-up chicken to the skillet and sauté until chicken is light golden and cooked through. Cover skillet and set aside.

COOKS' NOTE:

The leftovers can be stored in the refrigerator for up to 3 days in a tightly sealed container. Rewarm in the microwave.

* Although we like to use Newman's Own bottled dressings (they're of good quality and convenient), you can save money by making your own vinaigrette.

4. While the chicken is cooking, cook the pasta in a large pot of boiling water until tender. Drain the pasta; do not rinse it with cold water. Add the pasta to the skillet with the chicken and toss to combine. Scrape up the pan juices and cooked bits to mix into the pasta.

5. Pour the sauce mixture into the pasta and chicken and toss until well combined. Season with the salt and pepper, to taste. Spoon the pasta and chicken into the prepared baking pan. Top with the shredded Gruyère cheese and sprinkle with the nutmeg.

6. Place the baking dish in the center of the oven and bake at 375ºF for about 30 minutes, until golden brown and crisp on top. Serve immediately.

ASIAN NOODLES WITH CHICKEN

The fragrant aroma and subtle flavors of this noodle dish will entice you to make it over and over again. Rich and savory Asian elements take center stage: soy sauce, garlic, ginger, scallions, Chinese five-spice powder, hoisin sauce, and sesame oil. The sake adds a touch of sweet acidity to help round out the flavors. Take note: The dish can be vegetarian friendly if you make it with vegetable broth and tofu.

Serves 6

Marinade

2 tablespoons hoisin sauce

2 tablespoons sake

1 tablespoon soy sauce

1 tablespoon minced garlic

1 teaspoon sesame oil

1½ pounds boneless, skinless chicken breasts, thinly sliced

⅔ cup low-sodium chicken broth

2 tablespoons hoisin sauce

2 tablespoons soy sauce

2 tablespoons sake

1 tablespoon sesame oil

½ teaspoon Chinese five-spice powder

1 pound fettuccini

1 tablespoon canola oil

1 tablespoon minced fresh ginger

2 teaspoons minced garlic

3 ounces fresh baby spinach

½ cup chopped scallions

1. Make the marinade by combining the hoisin sauce, sake, soy sauce, garlic, and sesame oil in a medium-sized bowl. Toss the chicken with the marinade until the chicken is well coated. Cover and refrigerate overnight, or at least 2 hours.

COOKS' NOTE:
The leftovers can be stored in the refrigerator for up to 3 days in a tightly sealed container. Rewarm in the microwave.

2. Combine the chicken broth, hoisin sauce, soy sauce, sake, sesame oil, and Chinese five-spice powder in a large measuring cup. Heat the mixture in a small saucepan or in the microwave until hot and set aside.

3. Cook the pasta in a large pot of boiling water until tender. Drain the pasta; do not rinse it with cold water. Return the pasta to the pot.

4. While the pasta is cooking, heat the canola oil in a large, heavy skillet over medium-high heat (you can also use a large, heavy (5-quart) saucepan in order to avoid a lot of cleanup). Add the ginger and garlic and cook for 1 minute. Increase the heat to high and add the chicken; sauté until cooked through.

5. Add the cooked pasta and toss until pasta is coated. Add the warm sauce mixture, the baby spinach, and the scallions; toss until well combined. Turn off the heat, cover the skillet, and allow the pasta to sit for 3 to 4 minutes. Serve immediately.

PASTA WITH CREAMY GORGONZOLA AND MUSHROOM SAUCE

When you're looking for a pasta dish that's just a little different, our Creamy Gorgonzola and Mushroom Sauce is sure to please. We paired the richly pungent flavor of gorgonzola (use a good-quality cheese) with earthy mushrooms to create a satisfying dish with multiple layers of flavor. You can prepare it in 30 minutes or less, so it's perfect for a quick weeknight supper. Toss a big green salad and pour a hearty red wine to round out your meal.

Serves 4

2 tablespoons olive oil

2 tablespoons minced garlic

1 pound mushrooms, trimmed and sliced

2 cup canned diced tomatoes with liquid

2 tablespoons tomato paste

1 tablespoon dried basil

2 teaspoons dried oregano

1 cup crumbled Gorgonzola cheese

½ cup light cream

Salt and freshly ground black pepper

4 cups fusilli (spiral-shaped) or farfalle pasta

1. Heat the olive oil in a large, heavy skillet over medium heat. Add the garlic and cook 2 minutes, until golden. Add the mushrooms and sauté until they begin to soften, about 5 minutes. Add the tomatoes, tomato paste, basil, and oregano; bring to a simmer, lower heat, cover, and cook for 3 more minutes (sauce will thicken slightly). Add the Gorgonzola cheese and light cream; stir to blend. Season with the salt and pepper, to taste.

2. While the sauce is simmering, cook the pasta in a large pot of boiling water until tender. Drain the pasta; do not rinse it with cold water. Add the pasta to the skillet with the sauce. Cook over low heat for 2 minutes, so the pasta can absorb some of the sauce. Serve immediately.

COOKS' NOTE:
The leftovers can be stored in the refrigerator for up to 3 days in a tightly sealed container. Rewarm in the microwave.

PASTA WITH CHICKEN (OR SHRIMP) AND CREAMY PESTO SAUCE

It's easy to make pasta with pesto sauce, especially if you have some of the homemade variety tucked in the freezer. But a container of high-quality store-bought pesto will work just as well. Whichever you choose to use, here's an everyday pasta dish that is out of the ordinary. We've enriched it with quickly sautéed, marinated chicken, a touch of light cream, and some extra Parmesan cheese to create real comfort food that will nourish and calm your body. You can prep the chicken the night before and then come home and have dinner on the table in less than 30 minutes. This is a favorite pasta dish in our homes, and we believe it will become one in yours.

Serves 4

1 pound boneless skinless chicken breasts, thinly sliced (or 1½ pounds shrimp, peeled and deveined)

¼ cup Newman's Own Olive Oil & Vinegar Dressing*

2 teaspoons minced garlic

1 tablespoon olive oil

4 cups fusilli (spiral shaped)

1 cup frozen peas, thawed

¾ cup prepared pesto (use good-quality store-bought or homemade)

½ cup light cream (or heavy cream, optional)

½ cup grated Parmesan cheese

Salt and freshly ground black pepper

COOKS' NOTE:
The leftovers can be stored in the refrigerator for up to 3 days in a tightly sealed container. Rewarm in the microwave.

1. Place the chicken pieces and garlic in a medium-sized bowl and coat with the dressing. Cover and refrigerate overnight, or for at least 2 hours. (If using shrimp, use ¼ cup of the dressing and marinate for only 30 minutes.)

2. Heat the olive oil in a large, heavy skillet over high heat (you can also use a large, heavy 5-quart saucepan in order to avoid

* Although we like to use Newman's Own bottled dressings (they're of good quality and convenient), you can save money by making your own vinaigrette.

a lot of cleanup). Add the chicken (or shrimp) to the pan and sauté until cooked through.

3. While the chicken is cooking, cook pasta according to package directions and drain. Add the pasta to the skillet with chicken and toss to combine. Try to scrape up pan juices to mix into the pasta.

4. Add the peas, pesto, light cream, and Parmesan and stir until well combined; cook for 1 to 2 minutes, until the sauce is heated and a little can be absorbed by the pasta. Season with the salt and pepper, to taste. Turn off the heat; cover the pan and allow the pasta to sit for 3 to 4 minutes. Serve immediately.

MACARONI AND CHEESE

Nothing says comfort food like mac and cheese, but good gluten-free versions are hard to come by. Ours is based on the classic, time-tested recipe loved by kids big and small. It features a simple milk- and potato starch-based roux, enhanced with extra-sharp cheddar cheese—but feel free to make your own additions and changes. Replace some or all of the cheddar with Asiago, Fontina, Swiss, Jarlsberg, goat, or mozzarella cheese. Enhance the flavor with Dijon mustard, red pepper flakes, or other spices. No matter how you make it, you'll end up with a winning combination that's sure to bring smiles all around your table.

Serves 4 as a main course and 6 as side dish

8 ounces gluten-free elbow macaroni

2 tablespoons unsalted butter

2 teaspoons potato starch

½ teaspoon dry mustard

1 cup milk (whole is best)

2½ cups (about 10 ounces) shredded extra-sharp cheddar cheese, divided

Salt and freshly ground black pepper

COOKS' NOTE:
The leftovers can be stored in the refrigerator for up to 3 days in a tightly sealed container. Rewarm in the microwave.

1. Preheat the oven to 350°F. Place the rack in the center of the oven. Grease a 1-quart baking dish with cooking spray.

2. Cook the macaroni in a large pot of boiling water until tender. Drain the macaroni; do not rinse it with cold water.

3. While the macaroni is boiling, melt the butter in a medium-sized, heavy saucepan over low heat. Mix the potato starch and dry mustard into the melted butter and cook slowly, stirring constantly for 1 minute (the mixture will be bubbly and won't look like a traditional roux). Gradually stir in the milk. Increase the heat to medium and cook, stirring constantly, until the white sauce is smooth, thick, and reaches the boiling point.

4. Reduce the heat and add 2 cups of the shredded cheese. Stir until the cheese is melted. Spoon the sauce into the macaroni and stir until well combined. Add the salt and pepper, to taste.

5. Spoon the macaroni and cheese into the prepared baking dish. Top with the remaining ½ cup shredded cheese.

6. Place the baking dish in the center of the oven and bake at 350°F for about 20 to 30 minutes, until golden brown and crisp on top. Serve immediately.

RISOTTO

Risotto is versatile: We make it for a quick weeknight dinner and when we have dinner parties. We love to serve it year-round as a flavorful accompaniment to meat, poultry, or fish; a main course after a lush green salad; or sometimes as the first course before a light main entrée. We enjoy the flexibility risotto offers, because you can reach into your pantry and refrigerator, see what you have, and create a rich, nourishing dish that will sooth and satisfy everyone who eats it. Below we offer three of the most requested risottos in our own homes—a sophisticated, yet simple to make, Butternut Squash and Sage Risotto, a kid-pleasing Pepperoni Pizza Risotto, and a savory Risotto Carbonara that is more than a little addictive. You can also use our base recipe and substitute the cheese, vegetables, meat, herbs, and/or broth to create your own favorites.

Butternut Squash and Sage Risotto

Serves 4 as a main course; 6 as a side dish

½ cup pine nuts

½ cup freshly shredded Parmesan cheese

4 tablespoons milk

1 pinch freshly ground nutmeg

4–5 cups low-sodium vegetable broth (or low-sodium chicken broth)

2 tablespoons olive oil

1 cup finely chopped leeks, white parts and 1 inch of green parts (see Cooks' Note)

1 teaspoon minced garlic

2 tablespoons chopped fresh sage

1½ cups arborio rice

2 cups butternut squash flesh, finely diced

Salt and freshly ground black pepper

1. Toast the pine nuts in a small frying pan over medium heat until golden brown. In a food processor, combine the pine nuts, cheese, milk, and nutmeg until smooth. Set aside.

2. In a medium saucepan, bring the broth to a low simmer and keep it simmering.

3. Heat the oil in a 4-quart saucepan over medium heat and sauté the leeks, garlic, and sage for about 5 minutes, until the leeks are golden.

4. Add the rice and squash and sauté for 2 minutes, until all the rice grains are well coated, glistening, and semitranslucent.

5. Add 1 cup of the broth and simmer, stirring until absorbed. Continue to add the broth ½ cup at a time, stirring frequently, for about 20 to 25 minutes, until the rice is creamy. Reduce the heat, if necessary, to keep the fluid from being absorbed too quickly.

6. When there is only a small amount of liquid left in the risotto, stir in the nut and cheese mixture. Continue to simmer until all the liquid is absorbed.

7. Season with the salt and pepper, to taste. Cover the saucepan and let the dish rest for 2 minutes; serve immediately.

COOKS' NOTES:
To wash leeks: Cut off tops and then cut leek in half before washing out grit and sand.

The leftovers can be stored in the refrigerator for up to 3 days in a tightly sealed container. Rewarm in the microwave.

Pepperoni Pizza Risotto

Serves 4 as a main course; 6 as a side dish

4–5 cups low-sodium chicken broth

2 tablespoons unsalted butter

1 tablespoon olive oil

⅓ cup finely minced onion

1 teaspoon minced garlic

1½ cups arborio rice

½ cup dry white wine

3 ounces mozzarella, cut into cubes (fresh mozzarella is best)

¼ cup freshly grated Parmesan cheese

12 small, thin slices pepperoni, each slice cut in half

¼ cup prepared pizza sauce

¼ teaspoon dried oregano

Freshly ground black pepper

1. In a medium saucepan, bring the broth to a low simmer and keep it simmering.

2. Heat the butter and oil in a heavy 4-quart saucepan over medium heat. Add the onions and garlic and cook until softened (not browned), about 2 minutes, stirring occasionally.

COOKS' NOTE:
The leftovers can be stored in the refrigerator for up to 3 days in a tightly sealed container. Rewarm in the microwave.

3. Add the rice and stir until it is well coated, glistening, and semi-translucent, for 1 to 2 minutes. Add the white wine and stir until all the wine is absorbed. Add ½ cup of the hot broth and stir until the rice has absorbed most of the broth. Continue adding the broth, ½ cup at a time, and stir until all the broth has been absorbed. This should take about 20 more minutes. Reduce the heat, if necessary, to keep the fluid from being absorbed too quickly. The rice should be tender, but firm to the bite.

4. Add the mozzarella, Parmesan, pepperoni, pizza sauce, and oregano. Stir to combine with the rice and to heat the cheese and pepperoni. Season with the pepper, to taste. Cover the saucepan and let rest for 2 minutes; serve immediately.

Risotto Carbonara

Serves 4 as a main dish; 6 as a side dish

    4–5 cups low-sodium chicken broth

    2 tablespoons olive oil

    1 tablespoon unsalted butter

    2 teaspoons minced garlic

    ¼ cup minced shallots

    ⅓ cup diced hot Sopressata dry sausage

    1½ cups arborio rice

    ½ cup dry white wine

    1 tablespoon heavy cream

    1 tablespoon chopped fresh basil

    ⅛ teaspoon ground nutmeg

    ½ cup finely grated Parmesan cheese

    Salt and freshly ground black pepper

1. In a medium saucepan, bring the broth to a low simmer and keep it simmering.

2. Heat the olive oil and butter in a heavy 4-quart saucepan over moderate heat. Add the garlic and shallots and cook until softened (not browned), about 2 minutes, stirring occasionally.

3. Add the sausage and continue to cook until it browns around the edges, about 2 minutes, stirring occasionally.

4. Add the rice and stir until it is well coated, glistening, and semi-translucent, for 1 to 2 minutes. Add the white wine and stir until all the wine is absorbed. Add ½ cup of the hot broth and stir until the rice has absorbed most of the broth. Continue adding the broth, ½ cup at a time, and stir until all the broth has been absorbed. This should take about 20 more minutes. Reduce the heat, if necessary, to keep the fluid from being absorbed too quickly. The rice should be tender, but firm to the bite.

5. Add the heavy cream, basil, nutmeg, and Parmesan. Stir to combine. Cover and remove from the heat. Season with the salt and pepper, to taste. Cover the saucepan and let rest for 2 minutes; serve immediately.

COOKS' NOTE:
The leftovers can be stored in the refrigerator for up to 3 days in a tightly sealed container. Rewarm in the microwave.

QUINOA AND BLACK BEAN SALAD

Quinoa (keen-wa) is native to South America. It was a staple of the diet of the ancient Incas—hence its nickname, "the mother grain." Quinoa is a mild, nutty-tasting grain packed with high-quality protein, fiber, and iron. It cooks quickly, has a fluffy texture, and is available organically grown, packaged, and sold in natural food markets and many grocery stores. Quinoa is also a dietician's dream: One-third cup of dry quinoa has 160 calories, 3 grams of fiber, 6 grams of protein, and 20 percent of your daily requirement for iron and phosphorus. We decided to give quinoa a try. Our recipe is delicious served with grilled meats, poultry, or seafood.

Serves 6 as a side dish

1 cup quinoa

2 cups water

1 tablespoon olive oil

4 teaspoons fresh lime juice

½ teaspoon ground cumin

½ teaspoon ground coriander

2 tablespoons finely chopped fresh cilantro

2 tablespoons scallions

1½ cups cooked black beans (15-ounce can, drained)

1 cup diced tomatoes

1 cup diced roasted red pepper

1 tablespoon fresh green chilies

Salt and freshly ground black pepper

COOKS' NOTE:
The leftovers can be stored in the refrigerator for up to 3 days in a tightly sealed container. Rewarm in the microwave.

1. Put the quinoa in a sieve and rinse well under cool running water.

2. Bring the water to a boil in a medium-sized saucepan. Add the quinoa, cover, and simmer on low heat for 10 to 15 minutes, or until all of the water is absorbed and the quinoa is tender. Allow it to cool for 15 minutes.

3. In a large bowl, combine the oil, lime juice, cumin, coriander, cilantro, and scallions.

4. Stir in the beans, tomatoes, red peppers, and chilies. Add the cooled quinoa. Season with the salt and pepper, to taste, and combine thoroughly. Refrigerate until ready to serve.

Variation

- Leave out the black beans and substitute 1 pound of cleaned and deveined shrimp (tails removed) quickly sautéed in olive oil in a hot frying pan.

PESTO BRIE PIZZA WITH JALAPEÑO PEPPERS

We love to serve this delectable pizza as an hors d'oeuvre with wine, but it would also make an excellent main course after a salad. We top a prepared pizza crust with homemade or store-bought pesto, sliced Brie, and fresh jalapeño peppers and bake it until it's hot and a bit crisp. If you don't feel like slicing up Brie and jalapeños, you can make it in a hurry with pesto and shredded Pepper-Jack cheese for a similar effect. Although we love to use the homemade pizza crust recipe that follows, you can put the toppings on corn tortillas and cook them in a hot, well-greased frying pan for an even quicker version.*

Yields one 12-inch-round pizza or two 9-inch pizzas

1 prepared 12-inch pizza crust or 2 prepared 9-inch pizza crusts (recipe follows)
⅓ cup basil pesto
1 pound Brie cheese, rind removed, thinly sliced (1½ cups)
2 fresh jalapeño peppers, seeded and sliced thin

1. Place the rack in the lower third of the oven. Preheat the oven to 425ºF.

2. Put the pizza crust on a pizza pan (see the crust recipe that follows for pan specifications). Spread the pesto evenly over the prepared crust, leaving a ½-inch rim. Arrange the Brie evenly over the pesto. Arrange the jalapeño peppers evenly over the Brie.

3. Place the pizza pan on the center of the oven rack and bake at 425ºF for 10 minutes (8 minutes for a 9-inch crust). Remove the pizza from the pan and place it directly on the oven rack for 6 more minutes (4 minutes for a 9-inch crust). Remove the pizza from the oven and let it rest for 3 minutes. Slice and serve.

*To make more than one corn tortilla pizza at once, bake several on a large baking sheet in the bottom of an oven preheated to 425ºF (be sure to brush the baking sheet with olive oil first).

Pizza Crust

This crust is a classic New York-style thin crust, but you could make it thicker by baking it in a smaller pan (but be sure to adjust the baking time). Ideally, try to make the crust several hours or the day before you plan to use it. This gives the xanthan gum time to set, and the crust will be crisp and chewy—just like one made with wheat. If you make the crust just before you use it, it will still be delicious and the texture will still be wonderful, but the crisp and chewy aspect won't be as pronounced. Prebaked crusts freeze well, so you can make several and store them in the freezer.

Makes 1 12-inch-round pizza or 2 very thin 9-inch-round pizzas (recipe can be doubled)

Corn meal, optional

1 cup Brown Rice Flour Mix (see the Baking Appendix F, page 286)

½ cup millet flour (see the Baking Appendix F, page 286)

1 teaspoon xanthan gum

½ teaspoon salt

2 teaspoons granulated sugar

1 (¼-ounce) packet dry yeast granules (not quick-rise)

1 teaspoon olive oil

¾ cup plus 1 tablespoon water, heated to 110°F

1. Generously grease the pizza pan(s) or the bottom of the springform pan(s) with cooking spray. Lightly sprinkle the corn meal over the entire pan (optional). See Cooks' Note on the following page for pan specifications.

2. Mix together all the dry ingredients in a large mixing bowl with an electric mixer. Pour the olive oil and water into the mixing bowl and mix until just blended. Scrape the bowl and beaters, and then beat at high speed for 2 minutes.

3. Spoon the dough into the center of the prepared pan(s). Use a cake spatula to move the dough from the center to the outer rim of the pan using individual strokes; lightly dampen the

COOKS' NOTES:
This pizza crust can be prepared in advance: Precook the crust according to the directions, but do not put on the toppings. Remove from the oven and allow the crust to cool on a rack. Wrap well in plastic wrap and then foil; you may store it in the refrigerator for up to 2 days or the freezer for up to 3 weeks. Defrost the crust before using.

Dry ingredients can be mixed ahead of time and stored in plastic containers for future use. Do not add the yeast until just ready to bake the pizza.

COOKS' NOTE:

Pan specifications: Use 9-inch or 12-inch round pizza pans with ridged, and not smooth, bottoms. Sometimes, we use inexpensive foil pizza pans from the grocery store—or you can use the 12- or 9-inch bottom of a springform pan with a ridged, and not smooth, bottom. These pans are available from The Baker's Catalogue from King Arthur Flour (800-827-6836 or bakerscatalogue.com), Amazon.com, Sur La Table, other online sellers, and local kitchen supply stores. We prefer using the bottoms from inexpensive springform cake pans—we like the Kaiser brand, which has ridged, quilt-like bumps, just like the foil pizza pans. The bumps make the crust a little crisper and make it easier to spread the dough. If you can't find pans with ridges or bumps, use flat-bottomed ones. Your pizza will still be delicious.

spatula with warm water, as necessary. Try to arrange the dough so it covers the entire pan in a thin, even layer. Cover with a very light cloth and let rise in a warm place for 30 to 40 minutes. The pizza crust should approximately double in height.

4. Place the rack in the lower third of the oven. Preheat the oven to 425°F while the pizza is rising.

5. Bake the pizza in a pan on the rack of the preheated oven at 425°F for 15 to 16 minutes (12 to 14 minutes for a 9-inch pizza). The pizza should be light golden in color and cooked through. Remove from the oven and proceed with your pizza recipe.

For a softer crust:
Put on the pizza toppings and bake in the pan at 425°F for 15 to 20 minutes, or until the topping is cooked.

For a very crisp crust:
Put on the pizza toppings, remove the pizza from the pan, and place the pizza directly on the rack in the lower third of the oven. Bake at 425°F for 8 to 10 minutes (5 to 8 minutes for 9-inch pies), until the topping is cooked and the bottom is crispy.

To use a pizza stone:
Heat the stone according to the manufacturer's directions and place the prebaked crust, with any toppings, on the preheated stone. Bake at 425°F for 8 to 10 minutes, until the crust is crisp and the topping is cooked.

SESAME OATMEAL ROLLS

Give your eating habits a healthy and delicious twist with our Sesame Oatmeal Rolls. Fresh, hot gluten-free rolls take less time and effort to make than their wheat-containing counterparts: you just mix up the ingredients, scoop the dough into a cupcake pan, let them rise, and then into the oven they go. In less than an hour and a half, you can have the delicious comfort of a whole-grain roll on your table. Ours are enriched with oatmeal, sesame seeds, and omega-rich flax seeds, and they're perfect for eating alongside your favorite winter soups and stews. We also like to use them to make small sandwich rolls for breakfast with eggs and cheese, or for after-school snacks coated with peanut butter, banana, and locally harvested raw honey. (To rewarm the rolls for this purpose, first place them in the microwave for 15 seconds and then lightly toast them.) These delicate, slightly chewy rolls are easy to make and so delicious, you'll want to keep extra in the freezer so you can enjoy them all week long.

Makes 12 rolls

    Corn meal

    ⅓ cup gluten-free quick-cook or rolled oats

    2⅔ cups Bread Flour Mix A (see the Baking Appendix F, page 286)

    ¼ cup granulated sugar

    1 tablespoon flax seeds

    1 tablespoon toasted sesame seeds

    2 teaspoons xanthan gum

    1½ teaspoons salt

    1 (¼-ounce) packet dry yeast granules (not quick-rise)

    1½ cups water (heated to 110°F)

    2 teaspoons olive oil

    Additional sesame seeds, for sprinkling

1. Grease a 12-cupcake baking pan with cooking spray and sprinkle with the corn meal.

2. Lightly grind the oatmeal in a blender or small food processor to form a coarse flour. Mix all the dry ingredients in a large bowl with an electric mixer. Add the warm water (110°F) and olive oil to the bowl; mix until just blended. Scrape the bowl and beaters, and then beat at high speed for 2 minutes.

3. Scoop the dough for the rolls into the prepared cupcake pan with an ice cream scoop.

Dry ingredients can be mixed ahead of time and stored in plastic containers for future use, but do not add the yeast until you are ready to bake the bread.

Rolls can be stored in the refrigerator for up to 2 days or the freezer for up to 3 weeks; wrap well in plastic wrap and then foil. Refresh the rolls with a sprinkle of water and rewarm them in a 350°F pre-heated oven; wrap them in foil if you do not want a crisp crust (but open the foil for the last 5 minutes of reheating time).

Cover with a light cloth and let rise in a warm place (about 80°F) for 40 to 50 minutes, until the dough has slightly more than doubled in size.

4. Place the rack in the center of the oven. Preheat the oven to 400°F while the bread is rising. (Do not use a convection oven, because it will brown the rolls too quickly.)

5. Lightly coat the tops of the rolls with cooking spray (this will help the rolls brown slightly) and sprinkle with the additional sesame seeds. Bake for 15 to 25 minutes. The rolls should have a hollow sound when tapped on the sides and be light golden in color. An instant-read thermometer should register about 205 to 215°F. You can bake them longer to make a thicker crust; if you do, the color will deepen and the internal temperature will continue to rise. Remove the rolls from the pan and cool them on a rack.

BUCKWHEAT PANCAKES

Buckwheat pancakes are a hearty and delicious breakfast treat that is popular all over the country. At almost every baking class we teach, someone asks for a gluten-free buckwheat pancake recipe. This recipe always satisfies and is perfect with warm maple syrup and the Sunday paper. You can also create a tasty hors d'oeuvre with this recipe by making mini-pancakes topped with savory smoked salmon and fresh dill or caviar and sour cream (blinis).

Makes 8 pancakes

⅔ cup Brown Rice Flour Mix (see the Baking Appendix F, page 286)

⅓ cup buckwheat flour

¼ cup powdered buttermilk

1 teaspoon granulated sugar

2 teaspoons baking powder

½ teaspoon baking soda

½ teaspoon xanthan gum

¼ teaspoon salt

1 cup water

2 tablespoons canola oil

1 large egg, well beaten

½ teaspoon pure vanilla extract

Butter or canola oil, for greasing

1. Preheat a large, heavy skillet over medium-low heat.

2. Combine the dry ingredients in a medium-sized bowl and mix with a whisk. In a separate bowl, mix together the water, canola oil, egg, and vanilla, and then add the mixture to the dry ingredients. Mix gently until all ingredients are moist. The batter will be lumpy.

3. Brush the skillet with the butter or canola oil. Pour the batter (by ¼ cupful) into the heated skillet. Turn the pancakes when the bubbles on the top surface of the pancakes start to pop.

COOKS' NOTE:
Keep little bags of the recipe's premixed dry ingredients handy so you can quickly whip up a batch on a weekend morning.

4. Cook the pancakes about 1 to 2 minutes longer after turning and then remove them from the pan. (If the edges are flat when you cook them, the pan is too cool. If the pancakes brown before the little bubbles appear on the top and have time to pop, the pan is too hot.) Serve with your favorite syrup.

Variation

*   Add pecans, walnuts, or blueberries to the batter.

CLASSIC GRANOLA

Our classic granola is crunchy, not too sweet, and loaded with delicious fruit, nuts, seeds, coconut, honey, and spices. It stores well for months at a time, so you can make up a big batch to keep around the house. You can also give it away in beautifully tied packages as a present to your granola-loving friends. This recipe is simple to follow and so basic that you can also use it as a foundation for your own special additions. Enjoy it in small portions (¾ cup at a time) or sprinkle it on yogurt and fresh fruit. Either way, you'll be able to enjoy this scrumptious cereal any time you like.

Yields 12 cups

1 pound gluten-free quick-cook or rolled oats

1½ cups slivered raw almonds

1 cup coarsely chopped raw pecans

1 cup shredded unsweetened coconut

¾ cup flax seed meal

¾ cup raw sunflower seeds

1–2 teaspoons cinnamon (to taste)

½ teaspoon salt

¾ cup canola oil

¾ cup honey

8 ounces dried chopped dates, cranberries or other chopped dried fruit

1 cup Perky's Nutty Rice cereal, optional

1. Preheat the oven to 300°F. Position two racks in the top third and bottom third of the oven. Grease 2 large baking sheets with cooking spray.

2. Combine the oats, almonds, pecans, coconut, flax seed meal, and sunflower seeds in a large bowl. Sprinkle the cinnamon and salt over the top and stir.

3. Combine the oil and honey in a glass measuring cup and stir until combined; warm the mixture slightly in the microwave (or in a small saucepan) until the honey has melted. Pour over the granola mixture and mix well.

COOKS' NOTE:
Store in a tightly sealed container at room temperature for 2 weeks, in the refrigerator for 1 month, or the freezer for up to 3 months.

4. Divide the granola mixture between the 2 baking sheets and spread it out into a thin layer. Place the sheets in the oven and bake at 300°F for 20 to 25 minutes. Switch the placement of the baking sheets in the oven and stir the granola. Bake at 300°F for about 15 to 20 minutes more, until the granola is golden brown. Cool the granola on baking sheets and then spoon it back into the large bowl; mix in the dried dates or other dried fruit and the Nutty Rice cereal (if using).

CHAPTER 9

Fish and Seafood

Since the dawn of time, man has been catching fish to eat. But many people are hesitant about buying fish because it's so perishable. The freshest fish are ones you hunt (catch) yourself, but if you're like most of us gatherers, you need to find a reliable fishmonger. A quality fish market should have the sweet smell of prime seafood. The fish should be nestled in beds of shaved ice. Talk to your fishmonger to find out what kinds of fish are in season; those fish will be plentiful and less expensive.

THE SCIENCE OF PURCHASING SEAFOOD

Wild versus farm-raised seafood: Farm-raised seafood is commercially grown in tanks or enclosures in the ocean or in ponds, depending on the species. The fish are raised specifically to be sold for consumption—mostly by humans, but sometimes by animals. The fish don't have a lot of room to swim around and are more prone to disease than their sea-, lake-, and river-dwelling cousins. Therefore, antibiotics and pesticides are used in their production. Wild fish grow free of pesticides and antibiotics in their natural environment. They're also lower in fat, higher in protein, and contain more omega-3 fatty acids.

THE ART OF PURCHASING SEAFOOD

The art of purchasing seafood involves starting with the highest quality product. Buy fresh, or fresh-frozen, fish, and buy local whenever possible. Buy wild fish over farm raised when available.

Fresh fish should have a mild smell, whether you're buying it whole or in the form of a fillet or steak. The flesh should be moist, firm, and elastic, and it should have a fresh-cut appearance. There should be no leathery traces of yellowing or browning around the edges. When you buy a whole fish, the eyes should be clear and full, and not milky and sunken. The gills should be a bright reddish color.

When you buy frozen seafood, make sure it is frozen solid and that it doesn't have ice crystals or water stains. Do not buy it if there is an odor, any discoloration, or any type of drying, which can mean freezer burn.

For more detailed insights into the art and science of cooking seafood, review pages 68–75 in Chapter 4.

SHRIMP CURRY

Good curry dishes are notorious for requiring a lot of effort. Long lists of ingredients that require chopping, grinding, and roasting often put a dent in our desire to make them at home. But this Indian-style shrimp curry is fragrant and delicious, and it doesn't require hours of prep work in the kitchen. Serve it with basmati rice and some bright green vegetables for a well-balanced meal.

Serves 4

> 1½ pounds shrimp, peeled and deveined, with tails removed
>
> 2 tablespoons curry powder (make sure it's gluten free)
>
> 1 teaspoon ground coriander
>
> 1 teaspoon ground turmeric
>
> 4 tablespoons canola oil, divided
>
> 1 cup chopped onion
>
> 1 tablespoon minced peeled fresh ginger
>
> 1 tablespoon minced garlic
>
> 1 (13.5-ounce) can unsweetened coconut milk
>
> 1 cup low-sodium vegetable or chicken broth
>
> ½ cup canned crushed tomatoes
>
> 2 tablespoons chopped fresh cilantro
>
> Salt and freshly ground black pepper
>
> ½ teaspoon cayenne pepper, optional, if your curry is not hot enough
>
> Basmati rice, for serving

1. Put the shrimp in a small bowl. Mix together the curry powder, ground coriander, and turmeric in another small dish. Take 1 teaspoon of the spice mixture and add it to the shrimp with 1 tablespoon of the canola oil. Stir to coat all the shrimp and set aside to marinate for at least 15 minutes.

2. Heat 2 tablespoons of the canola oil in a large, heavy skillet over very high heat. Add the shrimp and quickly brown them on both sides, about 2 minutes total. Remove the shrimp to a small bowl and set aside.

3. Heat the remaining tablespoon of canola oil in the same skillet over medium-low heat. Add the onion, ginger, and garlic; cook until the onion is soft, about 4 minutes. Add the remaining curry powder, coriander, and turmeric mixture and sauté for about 1 minute. Stir in the coconut milk, broth, crushed tomatoes, and cilantro;

bring to a simmer and cover. Cook for 20 minutes over low heat, until the flavors are blended and the sauce has thickened slightly. Remove the cover and cook for another 10 minutes. Season with the salt and pepper, to taste. Add the shrimp and simmer for about 10 minutes (depending on size of shrimp) until shrimp is hot and cooked through. Add the cayenne pepper, if desired. Serve immediately with basmati rice.

Variation

- This dish can also be made with 1½ pounds of boneless, skinless chicken cut into 2-inch pieces in lieu of the shrimp.

SHRIMP PROVENÇAL

There are countless variations of this classic dish, but the foundation remains the same—quickly sautéed shrimp in a richly flavored sauce. Our version features canned tomatoes, although we like to use fresh when good ones are available at the end of the summer. Other than the shrimp, this is a dish you can throw together in minutes if you have a well-stocked pantry and a large skillet. It is really good with crusty French bread.

Serves 2–4

4 tablespoons extra virgin olive oil

1 pound large shrimp, shelled and deveined

2 shallots, minced

2 teaspoons minced garlic

3 tablespoons brandy

20 ounces canned diced tomatoes, with liquid

1 tablespoon tomato paste

1 teaspoon dried thyme

Salt and freshly ground black pepper

2 tablespoons chopped fresh parsley, for garnish

1. Heat the olive oil in a large, heavy skillet over medium-high heat. Add the shrimp and sauté until pink on both sides. Remove the shrimp from the pan.

2. Add the shallots and garlic to the pan and sauté over low heat until soft, about 3 to 4 minutes.

3. Turn off the heat and add the brandy. Turn on the heat to medium-high; stir to deglaze the pan and cook until the brandy is almost evaporated. Add the tomatoes, tomato paste, and thyme and bring to a boil. Simmer for 3 to 5 minutes. Add the shrimp back to the pan and cook until heated through, 1 to 2 minutes.

4. Remove from the heat. Season with the salt and pepper, to taste. Garnish with the parsley and serve immediately.

SOUTHWESTERN SHRIMP

This southwestern take on the classic Shrimp Provençal (see page 197) is sure to delight those around your table. It's a delectable dish that blends rich, smoky tomatoes and sweet crunchy shrimp with a touch of chipotle pepper for a little heat. The preparation is simple because we rely on a high-quality convenience product: a can of fire-roasted tomatoes (we recommend Muir Glen). Serve with freshly baked corn muffins and a salad of baby greens topped with your favorite dressing and some spicy pecans.

Serves 2–4

> 4 tablespoons extra virgin olive oil
>
> 1 pound large shrimp, shelled and deveined
>
> 2 shallots, minced
>
> 2 teaspoons minced garlic
>
> 3 tablespoons brandy
>
> 1 (14.5-ounce) can fire-roasted diced tomatoes with liquid*
>
> 1 tablespoon tomato paste
>
> 2 teaspoons molasses, optional
>
> 1 teaspoon minced canned chipotle pepper in adobo sauce
>
> 1 teaspoon dried oregano
>
> Salt and freshly ground black pepper
>
> 2 tablespoons chopped cilantro, for garnish

1. Heat the olive oil in a large, heavy skillet over medium-high heat. Add the shrimp and sauté until pink on both sides. Remove the shrimp from the pan.

2. Add the shallots and garlic to the pan and sauté over low heat until soft, about 3 to 4 minutes.

3. Turn off the heat and add the brandy. Turn on the heat to medium-high; stir to deglaze the pan and cook until the brandy is almost evaporated. Add the tomatoes, tomato paste, molasses (if using), chipotle pepper, and oregano and bring to a boil. Simmer for 3 to 5 minutes. Add the shrimp back to the pan and cook until heated through, 1 to 2 minutes.

4. Remove from the heat. Season with the salt and pepper, sprinkle with the cilantro and serve immediately.

*We recommend Muir Glen Organic Fire-Roasted Diced Tomatoes

SAUTÉED SEA SCALLOPS WITH CREAMY SHALLOT WINE SAUCE

Scallops are delicious and require relatively little effort to turn them into a special meal. This dish is quick and easy enough for a weeknight supper, but elegant enough to serve if you have guests. We like to pair it with colorful vegetables and a glass of white wine.

Serves 2

> ¾ pound sea scallops, rinsed and patted dry
>
> Salt and freshly ground black pepper
>
> 2 tablespoons butter
>
> ¼ cup white wine
>
> 2 tablespoons bottled clam juice
>
> 1 tablespoon minced shallots
>
> 2 tablespoons heavy cream

1. Season the scallops with salt and pepper, to taste. Heat the butter in a large, heavy skillet over high heat. Add the scallops and cook for 1½ minutes, until just firm and golden in color. Turn and cook the other side another 1½ minutes. Transfer scallops to a small bowl and cover with foil.

2. Add the wine, clam juice, and shallots to the skillet; scrape up the pan drippings. Boil until the liquid is reduced to a little less than ¼ cup. Stir in the heavy cream and add the scallops and any juices on the plate. Reduce the heat and cook another minute until the scallops and sauce are heated through. Serve immediately.

Variation

• Substitute fresh-squeezed lemon or orange juice for the heavy cream and then whisk in a little butter to make a smooth citrus butter sauce. Add chopped fresh herbs, such as basil or thyme.

STEAMED MUSSELS

Mussels are among the oldest known foods and can be found in cuisines around the world. Although this dish is more European in flavor, you can adapt it with herbs and spices to suit your own taste. Buy fresh mussels from a dependable fish seller and bring them home the same day to enjoy. Steamed mussels are easy to make for a fast, delicious weeknight supper with crusty bread, a big salad, and glass of white wine.

Serves 2–4

4 dozen mussels

2 tablespoons extra virgin olive oil

1 teaspoon minced garlic

2 shallots, minced

Zest of 1 lemon

Juice of 1 lemon

1 cup dry white wine

1 cup water

2 tablespoons chopped fresh herbs, such as basil, thyme, or dill

¼ cup chopped parsley

½ teaspoon salt

½ teaspoon freshly ground black pepper

1. Scrub the mussels and remove the beards. Discard any that do not close tightly. (A live mussel will remain rigidly closed. Discard any mussels if the shells partially open when you move them between your thumb and forefinger.)

2. Heat the olive oil in a large skillet over medium-high heat. Add the garlic and shallots and sauté over low heat for 5 minutes.

3. Add the lemon zest and juice, wine, water, herbs, parsley, salt, and pepper and bring to a boil. Simmer, covered for 2 minutes.

4. Add the mussels to the broth, cover the skillet, and then steam until all the mussels have opened, about 5 minutes.

5. Spoon the mussels and some broth into shallow bowls and serve hot.

Variation

- To make a red sauce: In Step 3, replace the wine with 1½ cups of fish stock or clam broth. Replace the water with 14.5 ounces canned diced tomatoes. Replace the lemon zest and lemon juice with ½ teaspoon of dried thyme. Simmer, covered, for 10 minutes. Continue with Step 4.

GRILLED AND ROASTED FISH FILLETS

Most of the fish we eat every week takes the form of simple-to-prepare grilled or roasted fillets. We have a few time-tested recipes that we turn to because they have become favorites for friends and family. Following is our short list—the recipes for grilling and roasting fish and the rubs, sauces, and various other toppings that form the basis of our fish cooking repertoire.

Basic Grilled Fish Fillet

Serves 4

> 1½ pounds fresh fish fillet (with skin or without skin), sliced 1 inch thick
>
> 1 tablespoon extra virgin olive oil
>
> Salt and freshly ground black pepper

1. Lightly grease the grilling surface (rack) with cooking spray. Preheat the grill to the high setting.

2. Brush the fillet with the olive oil and season with the salt and pepper, to taste; place on the greased rack (skin-side down, if applicable).

3. Grill for 5 minutes on the first side. Flip the fillet over. Grill for another 5 minutes on the other side. Remove immediately. Transfer to a serving plate (lift the fish from the skin, if applicable). Serve hot. As a general rule, allow 10 minutes total for each 1 inch of thickness on a hot grill.

Grilled Fish Fillet with Spice Rub

Serves 4

> 1½ pounds fresh fish fillet (with skin or without skin), sliced 1 inch thick
>
> 1 tablespoon extra virgin olive oil
>
> 1–2 tablespoons favorite spice rub

1. Lightly grease the grilling surface (rack) with cooking spray. Preheat the grill to the high setting.

2. Brush the top of the fillet with the olive oil and sprinkle with the spice rub to completely cover the entire surface; place on the greased rack (skin-side down, if applicable).

3. Grill for 10 minutes. Remove immediately and transfer to a serving plate (lift the fish from the skin, if applicable). Serve hot. As a general rule, allow 10 minutes total for each 1 inch of thickness on a hot grill.

Basic Roasted Fish Fillet

Serves 4

> 1½ pounds whole fresh fish fillet (with skin or without skin), sliced 1 inch thick
> 1 tablespoon extra virgin olive oil
> Salt and freshly ground black pepper

1. Place the rack in the center of the oven and preheat to 425ºF. Line a medium-sized heavy baking sheet with foil and lightly brush with olive oil.

2. Put the fillet on the baking sheet (skin-side down, if applicable) and brush the fillet with the olive oil. Season with the salt and pepper, to taste.

3. Place the baking sheet in the center of the oven and roast for 10 minutes per 1-inch thickness of the fillet. (If the fillet is 1½ inches, the roast time is 15 minutes.)

4. Remove from the oven and transfer to a serving plate (lift the fish from the skin, if applicable). Serve hot.

Roasted Fish Fillet with Spice Rub

Serves 4

> 1½ pounds whole fresh fish fillet (with skin or without skin), sliced 1 inch thick
> 1 tablespoon extra virgin olive oil
> 1–2 tablespoons favorite spice rub
> Juice 1 lemon (optional depending on rub)

1. Place the rack in the center of the oven and preheat to 425ºF. Line a medium-sized heavy baking sheet with foil and lightly brush with olive oil.

2. Place the fillet on the baking sheet (skin-side down, if applicable) and brush with the olive oil. Sprinkle with the spice rub to completely cover the entire surface.

3. Place the baking sheet in the center of the oven and roast for 10 minutes per 1-inch thickness of fillet. (If the fillet is 1½ inches thick, the roast time is 15 minutes.)

4. Remove from the oven (drizzle with fresh lemon juice, if desired) and transfer to a serving plate (lift the fish from the skin, if applicable). Serve hot.

ROASTED OR GRILLED FISH FILLET WITH TOMATO, CAPER, AND OLIVE TAPENADE

Serves 4

1. Roast or grill your fish according to the Basic Roasted Fish Fillet or Basic Grilled Fish Fillet recipes (see pages 201–202). Serve with Tomato, Caper and Olive Tapenade (recipe follows).

Tomato, Caper, and Olive Tapenade

> 2 tablespoons extra virgin olive oil
>
> 2 teaspoons minced garlic
>
> 2 cups diced canned tomatoes, drained (or fresh if good ones are available)
>
> ½ cup pitted chopped brine-cured black olives (such as Kalamata)
>
> 2 tablespoons capers
>
> Freshly ground black pepper

1. Heat the olive oil in a small, heavy saucepan over medium heat. Add the garlic and cook for 1 minute. Add the tomatoes, olives, and capers. Bring to a simmer and reduce the heat. Cook, uncovered, for about 5 minutes, until the tomatoes have wilted. Season with the pepper, to taste. Serve with roasted or grilled fish fillets.

ROASTED OR GRILLED FISH FILLET WITH RED PEPPER COULIS

Serves 4

1. Roast or grill your fish according to the Basic Roasted Fish Fillet or Basic Grilled Fish Fillet recipes (see pages 201–202). Serve with Red Pepper Coulis (recipe follows).

Red Pepper Coulis

> 1 tablespoon extra virgin olive oil
>
> ½ cup onions, finely chopped
>
> 2 large sweet red peppers, finely chopped, seeds and membranes removed
>
> 1 cup low-sodium chicken broth
>
> 2–3 tablespoons heavy cream or 2 tablespoons extra virgin olive oil
>
> Salt and freshly ground black pepper

1. Heat the olive oil in a heavy, medium-sized saucepan over medium-high heat. Add the onions and sauté until tender. Add the red peppers and chicken broth; bring to a boil. Simmer for 20 minutes and remove from the heat.

2. Place the red pepper mixture in a blender and purée until smooth. Pour the mixture back into the saucepan and boil until reduced to the thickness of heavy cream. Stir in the heavy cream or olive oil. Season with the salt and pepper, to taste. Serve with roasted or grilled fish fillets.

Variations

*   Add 2 teaspoons minced garlic.
*   Substitute 2 large yellow peppers for the red peppers.
*   Add ½ canned chipotle pepper (or to taste), chopped.
*   Add ½ fresh serrano chili (or to taste), chopped.

ROASTED OR GRILLED FISH FILLET WITH CITRUS BEURRE BLANC

Serves 4

1. Roast or grill your fish according to the Basic Roasted Fish Fillet or Basic Grilled Fish Fillet recipes (see pages 201–202). Serve with Citrus Beurre Blanc (recipe follows).

Citrus Beurre Blanc

  4½ teaspoons granulated sugar

  1½ teaspoons white wine vinegar

  1 cup orange juice

  3 tablespoons minced shallots

  ½ teaspoon minced garlic

  ½ cup dry white wine

  ½ cup fish stock*

  Juice of 1 lime

  2 tablespoons unsalted butter

  1 tablespoon chopped fresh cilantro

  Dash Tabasco sauce

  Salt and freshly ground black pepper

1. Put sugar and vinegar in a small saucepan and whisk to combine. Cook over medium-high heat until the sugar/vinegar mixture becomes a light caramel color.

2. Whisk in the orange juice and bring to a boil. Reduce the heat to medium and allow the mixture to reduce by half (about ½ cup), whisking occasionally. Set aside.

3. Combine the shallots, garlic, white wine, stock, and lime juice in a small sauté pan. Bring to a boil over medium-high heat until the mixture is reduced to ¼ cup of liquid. Whisk in the orange juice mixture and the butter. Stir in the cilantro and Tabasco sauce. Season with the salt and pepper, to taste.

4. Pour over the roasted or grilled fish fillets. Also delicious on sautéed scallops or shrimp.

* Can substitute low-sodium chicken broth, depending on the recipe.

ROASTED OR GRILLED FISH FILLET WITH DRY PASTRAMI RUB

Serves 4

1. Roast or grill your fish according to the Basic Roasted Fish Fillet with Spice Rub or Basic Grilled Fish Fillet with Spice Rub recipes (see pages 201–202).

Dry Pastrami Rub

> 3 tablespoons dark brown sugar
>
> 1 tablespoon ground coriander
>
> 1 tablespoon ground ginger
>
> 1 tablespoon garlic powder
>
> 1 tablespoon coarsely ground black pepper
>
> 1 tablespoon kosher salt
>
> 2 teaspoons paprika
>
> 1½ teaspoons allspice

1. Combine the dark brown sugar, coriander, ground ginger, garlic powder, pepper, salt, paprika, and allspice in a small, tightly sealed container. Store at room temperature or in the refrigerator.

ROASTED OR GRILLED FISH FILLET WITH FENNEL, ORANGE, AND ROSEMARY SPICED CRUST

Serves 4

1. Roast or grill your fish according to the Basic Roasted Fish Fillet with Spice Rub or Basic Grilled Fish Fillet with Spice Rub recipes (see pages 201–202).

Fennel, Orange, and Rosemary Spiced Crust

> 2 tablespoons fennel seed
>
> 2 tablespoons minced fresh rosemary
>
> 2 tablespoons minced fresh orange zest
>
> 1 teaspoon kosher salt
>
> ½ teaspoon freshly ground black pepper

1. Coarsely grind the fennel seeds in a spice grinder and mix with the rosemary, orange zest, salt, and pepper. Store in the refrigerator in a tightly sealed container for up to 1 week, or in the freezer for up to 1 month.

ROASTED OR GRILLED FISH FILLET WITH BLACK BEAN, CORN, AND TOMATO SALSA

Serves 4

1. Roast or grill your fish according to the Basic Roasted Fish Fillet or Basic Grilled Fish Fillet recipes (see pages 201–202). Serve with Black Bean, Corn, and Tomato Salsa.

Black Bean, Corn, and Tomato Salsa

1 (15.5-ounce) can black beans, rinsed and drained

¾ cup cooked fresh corn kernels or frozen corn kernels, thawed

3 medium plum tomatoes, chopped and seeded

4 medium scallions, thinly sliced

2 tablespoons chopped fresh cilantro

1 tablespoon red wine vinegar

1 teaspoon ground cumin

3 tablespoons extra virgin olive oil

Salt and freshly ground black pepper

1. Combine all above ingredients, except the salt and pepper, in a medium bowl and mix together. Season with the salt and freshly ground pepper, to taste.

OTHER FAVORITE FISH FLAVORINGS

- Sprinkle each fillet with dried thyme, dried dill, freshly ground black pepper, and coarse sea salt. Roast or grill your fish according to the Basic Roasted Fish Fillet or Basic Grilled Fish Fillet recipes (see pages 201–202).

- Add 1 teaspoon of curry powder to 1 tablespoon of extra virgin olive oil. Then brush flavored oil on the fish. Roast or grill your fish according to the Basic Roasted Fish Fillet or Basic Grilled Fish Fillet recipes (see pages 201–202). Before serving, sprinkle with Thai Ginger Sea Salt.*

- Sprinkle each fillet with Alderwood Fine Smoked Sea Salt* and freshly ground black pepper. Roast or grill your fish according to the Basic Roasted Fish Fillet or Basic Grilled Fish Fillet recipes (see pages 201–202).

* Gourmet flavored sea salts are available at specialty markets in jars or by the pound in the bulk area, and by mail order at http://www.saltworks.us/shop/category.asp?idCat=3. We recommend trying to buy the salts at your local market by the pound because it is much less expensive and a tablespoon lasts a long time. The ideas are endless. We even sprinkle the espresso flavored salts on homemade brownies.

GRILLED TAMARI-MARINATED SALMON

Fresh wild salmon is full of heart-healthy omega-3 fatty acids and vitamins A and D. We never tire of it and try to eat it every week. One of our favorite recipes is grilled tamari-marinated salmon. We like it because it is flavorful, simple to make, and incredibly versatile. Serve it with fresh seasonal vegetables and you can have dinner on the table in less than half an hour.

Serves 4

   1½ pounds fresh salmon fillets (1 inch thick) with skin

   ⅓ cup (gluten-free) tamari soy sauce

1. Place the salmon in a baking dish and pour the tamari soy sauce over the top and sides of the fish. Use a spoon to completely coat the fish's surface. Allow the fish to sit at room temperature for 1 hour.

2. Lightly grease the grilling surface (rack) with cooking spray. Preheat the grill to the high setting.

3. Grill the salmon fillet for 4 to 5 minutes, skin side down. Flip the fillet over, remove the skin and discard it. Grill for another 4 to 5 minutes on the other side. Remove immediately and serve. (Grill 8 minutes total if you like your salmon medium versus well cooked.)

Roasted Variation

- Add 2 teaspoons of minced ginger and 2 teaspoons of brown sugar to the tamari soy sauce. Marinate as described in Step 1. Roast skin-side down according to the Basic Roasted Fish Fillet recipe on page 202. Sprinkle 2 teaspoons of fresh lemon juice over fish just before serving.

- Marinate as described in Step 1. Prior to cooking, pat the top and sides of the salmon with 1 tablespoon of sesame seeds or Eden Shake Sesame and Sea Vegetable Seasoning Blend. Roast skin-side down according to the Basic Roasted Fish Fillet recipe on page 202.

Poultry and Meat Interlude

UNLIKE VEGETABLES, buying and purchasing poultry and meat is much more confusing. In an effort to simplify the process, we have tried to make sense of the more common labels. Understanding the terminology is both an art and a science.

THE SCIENCE OF COOKING POULTRY AND MEAT

Grass-Fed versus Grain-Fed

Grass-fed animals are pasture raised. There is no caging or confinement for these animals, and their diet consists of natural grasses, legumes, and plants. These animals are free of antibiotics, steroids, hormones, pesticides, and other foreign substances. Studies have shown that meat from pasture-raised animals is lower in fat and calories, contains more vitamin E, and is a richer source of conjugated linoleic acid (a good fat known to reduce cancer risks in humans), as compared to that of confined animals.[1] Grain-fed animals raised in confined feedlots are given diets specifically designed to fatten them up, which helps the farm boost its productivity and lower its costs. Genetically modified grain and soy are the main components of these animals' diets. To cut costs even more, animal feed may also contain such byproducts as municipal garbage, stale pastry, chicken feathers, and candy.

Organic

According to the 2001 USDA National Organic Program Consumer Brochure, organic food is

> produced by farmers who emphasize the use of renewable resources and the conservation of soil and water to enhance environmental quality for future generations. Organic meat, poultry, eggs, and dairy products come from animals that are given no antibiotics or growth hormones. Organic food is produced without using most conventional pesticides; fertilizers made with synthetic ingredients or sewage sludge; bioengineering; or ionizing radiation. Before a product can be labeled "organic," a Government-approved certifier inspects the farm where the food is grown to make sure the farmer is following all the rules necessary to meet USDA organic standards. Companies that handle or process organic food before it gets to your local supermarket or restaurant must be certified, too.[2]

Natural

A meat product labeled "natural" contains no artificial ingredients or added colors and is only minimally processed (a process which does not fundamentally alter the raw product). The label must explain the use of the term natural, such as "no added colorings or artificial ingredients" or "minimally processed." Unlike organic, the natural label does not require a certification process, and meat labeled natural may contain antibiotics. Federal regulations prohibit the use of hormones in raising pigs and poultry, but natural beef may contain hormones. Therefore, look for brands that are antibiotic and hormone free, with animals raised on a 100 percent vegetarian diet and no animal byproducts.

Free Range

Free range is a method of farming where the animals are allowed to roam free instead of being contained in any manner. It may apply to meat, egg, or dairy farming and does not mean that the animal was raised without antibiotics or hormones. Free-range chickens have access to the outdoors so that they can participate in activities similar to a natural environment. However, free range does not necessarily mean that the chickens actually venture outside, and if they do, the USDA mandate requires only 5 minutes of open-air time each day.

THE ART OF PURCHASING POULTRY AND MEAT

The art of purchasing poultry and meat involves starting with the highest quality product. Buy fresh, or fresh-frozen, meat or poultry, and buy locally raised products whenever possible. Buy meats and poultry that have been minimally processed and that contain no added saline solution, artificial coloring agents, preservatives, hormones, or antibiotics. Buy natural and grass-fed meat whenever possible. Buying organic is ideal. Fresh meat should be firm and should have a uniform color (beef and lamb should be red; pork is pink; and poultry is a pink/white color). The product should not have a brown or gray color or smell rancid.

Each of the recipes in the next two chapters will specify the recommended cut of meat or poultry that works best.

POULTRY AND MEAT INTERLUDE REFERENCES

1. Rule, D.C., K. S. Broughton, S. M. Shellito and G. Maiorano, (2002). "Comparison of Muscle Fatty Acid Profiles and Cholesterol Concentrations of Bison, Beef Cattle, Elk, and Chicken." *Journal of Animal Science* 80(5): 1202-11.

2. Gold, M.V. (2007). USDA National Agriculture Library. "Organic Production/Organic Food." USDA National Organic Program Consumer Brochure (2001). Accessed September 28, 2009 from http://www.nal.usda.gov/afsic/pubs/ofp/ofp.shtml.

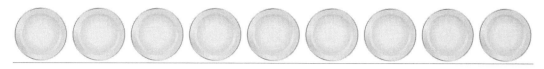

CHAPTER 10

Chicken and Turkey

Before you prepare any of the recipes in this chapter, consult the Poultry and Meat Interlude on pages 211–212 for insight on purchasing poultry with confidence. For more detailed insights into the art and science of cooking poultry, review pages 68–75 in Chapter 4.

Chicken Marsala

Chicken Paprikash

Thai Chicken

Mexican Chicken Tortilla Casserole

Chicken Pot Pie

    Traditional Pie Crust Dough

Corn Meal-Crusted Chicken

Chicken Parmesan

Chicken and Sausage Jambalaya

Grilled Chicken with Lemon, Rosemary, and Garlic

Turkey Cutlets

    Turkey Cutlet Piccata

    Turkey Cutlet Scaloppini

CHICKEN MARSALA

Chicken Marsala is a traditional Italian dish that dates back to the 19th century. When you make it with good-quality, fresh ingredients, you'll rediscover this flavorful old favorite. Our recipe blends sweet Marsala wine with savory mushrooms, shallots, and marjoram to create a dish of simple elegance. It is special enough to serve for a quiet Saturday night dinner with friends; just add pasta, sautéed vegetables, a scrumptious dessert, and a bottle of wine. The bonus is that you can cook it up in no time and serve it for a weeknight dinner anytime. We think it will become a new old favorite in your home.

Serves 4 as a main dish

¼ cup brown rice flour

1 teaspoon onion powder

1 teaspoon salt

¼ teaspoon black pepper

1½ pounds chicken cutlets (¼ inch thick)

3 tablespoons extra virgin olive oil, divided

1 teaspoon minced garlic

¼ cup minced shallots

1 teaspoon dried marjoram

½ pound mushrooms, thinly sliced

2 tablespoons unsalted butter, divided

¾ cup Marsala wine

½ cup low-sodium chicken broth

1 rounded teaspoon chicken demi-glace*

Salt and freshly ground black pepper

Cooked gluten-free pasta, for serving

1. Combine the brown rice flour, salt, pepper, and onion powder in a flat dish; dredge the chicken cutlets in the flour mixture.

2. Heat a large, heavy skillet over medium heat. Add 1 tablespoon of the olive oil and sauté the garlic and shallots until softened. Add the marjoram and mushrooms and sauté until the mushrooms release their juices. Remove from the pan and set aside in a small bowl.

*We recommend More than Gourmet brand.

3. Add another tablespoon of the olive oil and 1 tablespoon of the butter to the skillet and heat over medium-high heat. Brown the chicken cutlets on both sides in 2 or 3 small batches, adding the remaining oil and butter as necessary. Remove the chicken from the skillet and set aside on plate. Cover with foil.

4. Add the wine, broth, and demi-glace, stir to combine, and boil until the liquid is reduced to 1 cup (about 2 to 3 minutes). Return the chicken and mushrooms to the skillet, cover, and simmer over medium-low heat until the chicken is cooked through, about another 5 minutes. Season with the salt and freshly ground black pepper, to taste. Serve with fresh hot gluten-free pasta.

COOKS' NOTE:
Cook the mushrooms and prep the chicken cutlets ahead of time, so all you have to do is quickly sauté them while you cook the pasta. You can also finish cooking the dish earlier in the day and then reheat it when you are ready to serve (reheat in a large, covered skillet over low heat on the stove).

CHICKEN PAPRIKASH

We grew up in a community that had wonderful, family-owned, Hungarian restaurants. A much-loved dish when we were young was chicken Paprikash with spaetzle. This recipe is our tribute to those delicious meals. We combine rich, tart sour cream, sweet onions, and richly colored, vitamin C-rich paprika to make a robust dish that will satisfy everyone around the table. Although classic recipes use a cut-up whole chicken, we've streamlined our recipe for time-pressed cooks, but the chicken is still tender with our finely tuned cooking method. Serve it with buttered pasta and lots of fresh vegetables for a quick and hearty meal.

Serves 6

> 3 tablespoons canola oil, divided
>
> 2 pounds boneless skinless chicken breasts or thighs, cut into 2-inch pieces
>
> 1 cup minced onion
>
> 1 tablespoon sweet Hungarian paprika
>
> 1 cup low-sodium chicken broth
>
> 1 heaping teaspoon chicken demi-glace*
>
> 1 tablespoon potato starch
>
> 1 cup low-fat sour cream
>
> Salt and freshly ground black pepper
>
> Cooked buttered gluten-free pasta, for serving

1. Heat 2 tablespoons of the canola oil over high heat in a large, heavy skillet. Sauté half the chicken until golden brown on all sides. Remove to a plate and brown the remaining chicken. (Add more oil, if necessary.) When golden, remove to the plate with the other browned chicken.

2. Reduce the heat to medium and add the remaining tablespoon of canola oil. Sauté the onions until golden brown and tender. Add the paprika and stir, coating the onions.

3. Add the chicken broth and demi-glace; stir to combine. Return the chicken and any accumulated juices to the skillet. Increase the heat and bring to barely a simmer. Cover the pan, reduce the heat to low, and cook for 15 to 20 minutes, or until the chicken is tender and cooked through.

4. Stir the potato starch into the sour cream and add the mixture to the chicken and sauce; stir to combine. Season with the salt and pepper, to taste. Increase the heat and simmer, covered, for another for 2 minutes, or until heated through and thickened. Serve with fresh, hot, buttered gluten-free pasta.

*We recommend More than Gourmet brand.

THAI CHICKEN

This dish is comforting and fast—ready in less than 20 minutes. Our Thai inspired dish is the perfect solution to the cry, "Not chicken again!" Spice up the week and savor the flavor.

Serves 3–4

> 2 tablespoons canola oil
>
> 1 pound boneless, skinless chicken breasts, cut chicken into 2-inch thin strips
>
> 1 (14-ounce) can coconut milk
>
> 2 tablespoons red curry paste*
>
> 3 tablespoons fish sauce
>
> 1 tablespoon brown sugar
>
> 1 tablespoon chopped fresh basil
>
> ½ cup scallions, finely chopped
>
> ¼ cup chopped fresh cilantro
>
> Cooked rice, for serving

1. Heat the oil in a large, heavy saucepan over medium-high heat. Sauté the chicken strips until lightly browned, about 3 to 5 minutes. Stir in the coconut milk and red curry paste; simmer for 5 minutes.

2. Reduce the heat to medium-low and stir in the fish sauce, brown sugar, and basil. Cook for 5 minutes.

3. Remove from the heat. Sprinkle with the scallions and cilantro and serve hot over the rice.

*We recommend Thai Kitchen Red Curry Paste, available at most supermarkets.

MEXICAN CHICKEN TORTILLA CASSEROLE

Here is a classic Tex-Mex favorite made without the highly processed, canned soups that many home cooks rely on for their recipes. We make a lower-fat, chemical-free version with our Creamy Chicken Garlic Sauce Base. You can prep much of the casserole ahead of time (you can even buy a cooked rotisserie chicken) and then assemble it when you are ready to pop it in the oven for dinner.

Serves 4–6

2 small cans chopped green chilies (about 7 ounces total)

2½ cups Creamy Chicken Garlic Sauce Base (see page 85)

4 cups cooked boneless chicken, sliced into thin 2-inch strips

1 teaspoon dried oregano

1 teaspoon ground cumin

¼ cup chopped fresh cilantro

Salt and freshly ground black pepper

12 fresh corn tortillas

2½ cups grated cheddar cheese, divided

1. Preheat the oven to 350°F. Place the rack in the center of the oven. Grease a 2½- or 3-quart casserole dish with cooking spray.

2. Purée the green chilies with the Creamy Chicken Garlic Sauce Base in a blender and set aside.

3. Toss the sliced chicken with the oregano, cumin, and cilantro. Season with the salt and pepper, to taste.

4. Soften 4 tortillas between 2 sheets of damp paper towel in a microwave for about 45 seconds. Arrange the tortillas along the bottom and sides of the casserole dish (tortillas will overlap). Spoon half the chicken over the tortillas. Sprinkle with ¾ cup of the grated cheese, and then cover with half of the sauce.

5. Arrange a second layer of 4 overlapping tortillas over the sauce (do not presoften). Repeat layers of the chicken, cheese, and sauce. Top with a layer of 4 overlapping tortillas (do not presoften) and the remaining cheese. (Do not assemble until you are ready to bake).

6. Bake at 350°F for 45 minutes to 1 hour, until hot. Serve immediately.

Variation

• Add chopped olives, red pepper, or diced tomato to the chicken and spices before assembling.

CHICKEN POT PIE

We have childhood memories of the Swanson pot pies our mother served us when she and our father were going out for the evening. Over time, we still wanted to enjoy the old-fashioned comfort of a pot pie, but we wanted a fresher, less processed version. We created a recipe and then fine-tuned it so our pot pies take less time to make than you'd think—and they're so good that everyone in our families look forward to eating them, kids and grownups alike.

Our Creamy Chicken Soup Base provides a rich, flavorful sauce to which we add cooked chicken, vegetables, herbs, and other seasonings. The pie crust (recipe follows) is easy to prepare and makes a perfect topping for the pot pie. If you want to make this for a weeknight, you can prep the Soup Base and pie crust ahead of time and then quickly assemble the pie before you bake it.

Serves 5–6

> 3 generous cups russet potatoes, peeled and cut into bite-size pieces
>
> 1 cup carrots, cut into bite-size pieces
>
> 3 cups Creamy Chicken Soup Base (made with garlic) (see page 91)
>
> 1 rounded teaspoon chicken demi-glace*
>
> 1 tablespoon dry sherry
>
> 2 tablespoons fresh dill or 1 tablespoon dried dill
>
> 1 teaspoon dried thyme
>
> 1 cup frozen peas (defrosted)
>
> 4 generous cups cooked chicken, cut into bite-size pieces (about 1¾ pounds chicken before cooking)**
>
> ⅓ cup light cream
>
> Salt and freshly ground black pepper
>
> Traditional Pie Crust Dough (recipe follows)

1. Preheat the oven to 375°F. Place the rack in the center of the oven. Grease a large 9- to 10-inch round deep-dish pie pan or a 10-inch-round × 2½-inch-high baking dish with cooking spray.

2. Boil or steam the potatoes until fork tender. Set aside. Boil or steam the carrots until fork tender. Set aside.

---

*We recommend More than Gourmet brand.

**Here's a quick and easy method to cook the chicken: Place raw, cubed chicken in a large skillet. Turn the heat to medium, cover, and cook, stirring occasionally, until the chicken is cooked through, about 10 minutes. Drain the liquid from the skillet and add the chicken.

3. Put the Creamy Chicken Soup Base in a large, heavy saucepan. Add the demi-glace, sherry, dill, and thyme bring to a boil over medium-high heat. Remove from the heat and stir in the peas, chicken, potatoes, carrots, and light cream. Season with the salt and pepper, to taste.

4. Roll the pie crust dough between two sheets of waxed paper until the circle is large enough to cover the top of the pie pan, with about ½ to ¾ of an inch hanging over the side.

5. Pour the chicken mixture into the baking dish and top with the rolled pie crust dough. Crimp the pie crust dough around the edges of the pie pan to create a decorative border. Make 2 or 3 slits in the top of the pie to allow steam to release. Place in the center of the oven and bake for 40 to 45 minutes, or until the crust is light golden brown.

Traditional Pie Crust Dough

This is really a fabulous pie crust—perhaps even better than those made with wheat. It stands up well to fruit fillings, custards, and even lemon meringue. It is probably the only pie crust you will ever eat that is as good the second day as it is the first. It is easy to make in a mixer—no messy hands or time-consuming pastry cutters. You will become a pie crust-making phenomenon in your own home.

Makes one 8- or 9-inch pie crust or one 10-inch tart

1 cup plus 2 tablespoons Brown Rice Flour Mix (see the Baking Appendix F, page 286)

2 tablespoons sweet rice flour (see the Baking Appendix F, page 286)

1 tablespoon sugar

½ teaspoon xanthan gum

¼ teaspoon salt

6 tablespoons cold unsalted butter, cut into six pieces (not margarine)

1 large egg

2 teaspoons orange juice or lemon juice

1. Mix the flours, sugar, xanthan gum, and salt in the large bowl of an electric mixer. Add the butter and mix until the mixture is crumbly and resembles a coarse meal.

2.	Add the egg and orange juice. Mix on low speed until the dough holds together; it should not be sticky. Form the dough into a ball using your hands and place on a sheet of wax paper. Top with a second sheet of wax paper and flatten the dough to 1-inch thickness. *The dough can be frozen at this point for up to one month; wrap in plastic wrap and then use foil as an outer wrap on top of the plastic.*

6.	Roll out the dough between the 2 sheets of wax paper. If the dough seems tacky, refrigerate for 15 minutes before proceeding. Remove the top sheet of wax paper and invert the dough into a pie pan (or on top of a pot pie). Remove the remaining sheet of wax paper, and crimp the edges for a single crust pie. *If you are going to use the crust to make a regular pie, the dough can also be frozen after it is in the pie pan for up to 1 month; line the pie shell with wax paper, wrap in plastic wrap, and use foil as an outer wrap.*

To prebake a bottom pie crust:
Preheat the oven to 375ºF. Gently prick the pastry in 3 or 4 places with a fork. Bake the pastry for about 25 minutes or until golden. Remove from the oven and cool completely on a wire rack. *Prebaked pie shells can be stored in airtight plastic containers or plastic wrap in the refrigerator for 3 days. For longer storage, wrap in plastic wrap and then foil and store in the freezer for up to 2 weeks.*

To partially bake a bottom pie crust:
Preheat the oven to 375ºF. Bake the pastry for 10 minutes. Remove from the oven. Fill and bake as per recipe. Partially bake the pie crust whenever you are making a fruit pie or quiche.

CORN MEAL-CRUSTED CHICKEN

We like to make this fast and easy chicken dish on weeknights. The crisp, crunchy cutlets can be ready in less than 20 minutes and are delicious with ready-made salsa or chutney. Serve them alongside whatever vegetables you have on hand for a colorful, healthy dinner everyone will enjoy.

Serves 4

> 4 boneless, skinless chicken breasts (about 1½ pounds)
>
> ¼ cup brown rice flour
>
> 1 large egg, beaten
>
> ⅔ cup corn meal
>
> Salt and freshly ground black pepper
>
> 3 tablespoons canola oil
>
> Ready-made salsa or chutney, for serving

COOKS' NOTE:
See the following recipes in this book for healthy meal complements: Black Bean, Corn, and Tomato Salsa on page 208 and White Beans with Tomato and Red Onion on page 162. Or try the chicken with our Spicy Roasted Ratatouille Spread on page 138.

1. Place each chicken breast between 2 pieces of wax paper (or plastic wrap) and pound to ½-inch thickness with a meat mallet or rolling pin.

2. Place the brown rice, egg, and corn meal each in separate shallow dishes.

3. Sprinkle each breast with salt and pepper and dredge them lightly in the brown rice flour. Dip each breast in the beaten egg, coating completely. Dip and coat each breast in the corn meal. Place the breasts on a platter.

4. Heat the canola oil in a large, heavy skillet over medium heat. Place the chicken in the skillet and cook for about 2 to 3 minutes on each side, until the coating is crisp and the chicken is cooked through. Serve with salsa or chutney.

CHICKEN PARMESAN

Here is a tried and true version of an old classic. Filled with the rich, warm flavors of Italy, chicken Parmesan is easy enough to make on a week night, but delicious enough to serve to a weekend crowd. You can make it ahead and gently rewarm it covered with foil in a preheated 350°F oven. Enjoy your meal with pasta and a large green salad.

Serves 4

4 boneless, skinless chicken breasts (about 1½ pounds)

¼ cup brown rice flour

⅛ teaspoon black pepper

⅛ teaspoon salt

1 large egg, lightly beaten

¾ cup gluten-free bread crumbs*

1 teaspoon Italian seasoning

¼ cup grated fresh Parmesan cheese

1 tablespoon extra virgin olive oil

1½ cups favorite prepared tomato sauce

1 cup (4 ounces) shredded mozzarella cheese

1 cup (4 ounces) shredded provolone cheese

1 tablespoon chopped fresh parsley

1 tablespoon chopped fresh basil

1. Preheat the oven to 400°F. Place the rack in the center of the oven. Grease an 11- × 7-inch baking dish with cooking spray or brush with olive oil.

2. Place each chicken breast between 2 sheets of wax paper (or plastic wrap) and pound to ½-inch thickness with a meat mallet or rolling pin.

3. Combine the flour, pepper, and salt in a flat dish. Place the beaten egg in a shallow dish. Combine the bread crumbs, Italian seasoning, and Parmesan cheese in a shallow dish.

4. Dredge the chicken breasts in the flour and then dip them in the beaten egg. Next, dredge the breasts in the bread crumb mixture. Place the breasts on a platter.

* An economical, easy to make gluten-free bread crumb recipe is available in *Gluten-Free Baking Classics, Second Edition*, by Annalise Roberts (Surrey Books, 2008). You can also simply grind up the ends of a loaf of gluten-free bread in a blender or food processor and then bake the crumbs in the oven at 325°F until lightly browned.

5. Heat the oil in a large, heavy skillet over medium-high heat. Add the chicken and sauté for 1 to 2 minutes on each side or until golden brown. Remove from the heat.

6. Spread ½ cup of the tomato sauce in the prepared baking dish. Arrange the chicken breasts in a single layer on top of the sauce. Top each piece with ¼ cup of the sauce. Sprinkle with the mozzarella and provolone cheese.

7. Bake for 10 minutes, or until the cheese is melted and bubbling slightly. Sprinkle with the parsley and basil and serve immediately.

CHICKEN AND SAUSAGE JAMBALAYA

Put on some highly seasoned bayou country music and dish up a pot of our jambalaya for your next dinner party. The folks on the bayou have gathered together and shared jambalaya by the cast-iron-pot-full since the late 18th century. Think of jambalaya as spiced-up Spanish paella—Cajun style. Cajun cuisine blends the ingredients and techniques of French, German, Spanish, African and American Native influences with local bayou flavor. Cayenne replaces saffron in this flavorful festive dish in order to give it some heat. Jambalaya is perfect for entertaining because it is inexpensive to make, easy to prepare, and cooks all in one pot in just 40 minutes. So invite some friends over and cook up a pot full to share this weekend.

Serves 6–8

3 tablespoons canola oil

2 pounds boneless, skinless chicken breasts (or thighs), cut into 2-inch pieces

4 cups chopped onion

1 cup chopped green pepper

1 tablespoon minced garlic

1 pound Creole smoked sausage (if unavailable, look for smoked Polish or French garlic sausages), cut into ½-inch pieces

3 tablespoons chopped fresh, or 1 tablespoon dried, parsley

2 teaspoons salt

2 whole bay leaves, crushed

½ teaspoon freshly ground black pepper

½ teaspoon chili powder

¼ teaspoon dried thyme

¼ teaspoon dried basil

¼ teaspoon cayenne or crushed red pepper

⅛ teaspoon crushed cloves

1 cup baked ham, chopped into bite-size pieces

1½ cups uncooked long-grain rice

3 cups water

1. Heat 2 tablespoons of the oil in a large, heavy (6- to 7-quart) saucepan over high heat. Add the chicken and brown on all sides. Remove to a bowl and set aside.

2. Add 1 tablespoon of the oil to the pot and lower the heat to medium. Add the onion, green pepper, and garlic; cook, stirring frequently, until the vegetables are softened

COOKS' NOTE:

If using chicken thighs, add the chicken to the pot after 10 minutes (instead of 15 minutes). Push the thighs down into the rice and cook about 20 minutes longer, until the chicken is cooked through.

and slightly browned, about 5 minutes. Add the sausage, parsley, salt, bay leaves, black pepper, chili powder, thyme, basil, cayenne pepper, and cloves; continue cooking and stirring for 5 minutes. Add the ham and stir 1 minute more.

3. Add the rice and stir until well combined. Add the water and stir while scraping the bottom of the pot. Increase the heat to high, cover, and bring to a full boil. Stir well, reduce the heat to low, and cook for 15 minutes. Add the chicken to the pot (do not add any juices from the bowl) and stir, pushing the chicken down into the rice. Cook for 15 minutes more, stirring occasionally, until the chicken is cooked through and the liquid is absorbed. Remove from heat and allow to rest 5 minutes.

GRILLED CHICKEN WITH LEMON, ROSEMARY, AND GARLIC

This recipe makes our top-ten list and is our favorite way to serve grilled chicken. It requires very little in the way of preparation, but the result is tender, flavorful chicken every time. It makes a delicious outdoor meal when served with grilled vegetables, a colorful bean salad (try our White Beans with Tomato and Red Onion recipe on page 162), and some crusty rustic flat bread.*

Serves 6

½ cup Newman's Own Olive Oil & Vinegar Dressing**

¼ cup fresh lemon juice

3 tablespoons chopped fresh rosemary

1 tablespoon grated fresh lemon zest

2 teaspoons minced garlic

Freshly ground black pepper

2 pounds boneless, skinless chicken breasts, cut in half

1. Combine the dressing, lemon juice, rosemary, lemon zest, garlic, and pepper in a large bowl and mix well.

2. Place the chicken in a bowl and toss to coat with the marinade. Cover and refrigerate for at least 4 hours (overnight is best), turning occasionally.

3. Preheat and prepare the barbecue. Grill the chicken over medium heat, basting occasionally with the marinade. Cook for 15 to 20 minutes, or until done, turning every 5 minutes. Transfer to a clean serving platter and serve hot.

* A gluten-free rustic flat bread recipe is available in *Gluten-Free Baking Classics, Second Edition*, by Annalise Roberts (Surrey Books, 2008).

** Although we like to use Newman's Own bottled dressings (they're of good quality and convenient), you can save money by making your own vinaigrette.

TURKEY CUTLETS

Turkey cutlets make healthy meals that are quick and easy and perfect for family dining. They can be paired with wine, broth, and a bountiful variety of herb and spice combinations to make interesting, flavorful dishes. Below are two savory classics we make all the time. However, these recipes are easy to adapt and lend themselves to change. For an Asian flair, try soy sauce, honey, and a hint of orange juice. For a more rustic version, substitute the lemon, capers, and parsley for fresh sage and heavy cream.

Turkey Cutlet Piccata

Serves 4

> 1¼ pounds turkey cutlets
>
> Salt and freshly ground black pepper
>
> 3 tablespoons brown rice flour
>
> 1 tablespoon olive oil
>
> 1 tablespoon unsalted butter
>
> ¼ cup white wine
>
> 1 tablespoon fresh lemon juice
>
> 1 tablespoon small capers
>
> 1 tablespoon chopped fresh parsley

1. Pat the cutlets dry, sprinkle with salt and pepper, and dredge lightly in the rice flour.

2. Heat the olive oil and butter in a large, heavy skillet over medium-high heat. When hot, sauté the turkey cutlets until lightly browned and cooked through, about 2 to 3 minutes per side. Remove to a platter and cover with foil to keep warm.

3. Add the wine, lemon juice, and capers to the skillet and bring to a boil, scraping up any browned bits. Add the parsley and season with more salt and pepper, to taste. Arrange cutlets on serving plates and pour the sauce over the top. Serve hot.

Turkey Cutlet Scaloppini

Serves 4

1¼ pounds turkey cutlets

Salt and freshly ground black pepper

3 tablespoons brown rice flour

2 tablespoons olive oil

1 tablespoon unsalted butter

2 teaspoons minced garlic

2 bay leaves

2 tablespoons cognac or brandy

½ cup low-sodium chicken broth

1 tablespoon chopped fresh parsley

2 tablespoons heavy cream, optional

1. Pat the cutlets dry, sprinkle with salt and pepper, and dredge lightly in the rice flour.

2. Heat the olive oil and butter in a large, heavy skillet over medium-high heat. Add the garlic and bay leaves, cook for 1 minute, and add the cutlets. Sauté the cutlets for 2 to 3 minutes per side until golden brown and cooked though. Remove the bay leaves and discard them. Remove the cutlets to a platter, and cover them with foil to keep warm.

3. Turn off the burner and add the cognac to the skillet; deglaze the pan by scraping up any browned bits. Turn the burner back on, add the broth, and bring to a boil; simmer for 2 minutes, until slightly reduced. Add the parsley and heavy cream (if using). Season with more salt and pepper, to taste. Arrange the cutlets on serving plates and pour the sauce over the top. Serve hot.

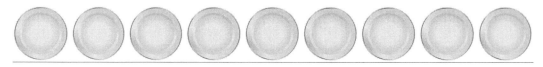

CHAPTER 11

Meat

Before you prepare any of the recipes in this chapter, consult the Poultry and Meat Interlude on pages 211–212 for insight on purchasing meat with confidence. For more detailed insights into the art and science of cooking meat, review pages 68–75 in Chapter 4.

Beef Stroganoff

Beef Stir-Fry with Oyster Sauce

Southwestern Braised Chuck Roast

Brisket with Barbecue Sauce

Grilled Beef Fillet Steaks with Garlic Paste

Sautéed Pork with Maple Mustard Sauce

Pork with Apples and Calvados

Slow-Braised Pulled Pork

    Red Bean Sauce

Grilled Pork Tenderloin Teriyaki

Baby-Back Ribs with Southern Spice Rub

    Southern Spice Rub

Pork Tenderloin with Southern Spice Rub

Grilled Pork Tenderloin with Ancho–Chipotle Chili Marinade and Black Bean Sauce

    Black Bean Sauce

Roasted Leg of Lamb with Garlic Crust

Moroccan Lamb (or Chicken) Stew

Grilled Tandoori Lamb with Cucumber Raita

    Cucumber Raita

Buffalo Meatballs

Veal Meatball Stroganoff

BEEF STROGANOFF

Beef Stroganoff is a seemingly dramatic dish that you can count on to make the people around your table happy. Special enough for a dinner party, but simple enough to whip up on a weeknight, the savory aroma and rich beef flavor combine to make this a dish we love to serve any time of year.

Serves 8–10

1 tablespoon canola oil

3 tablespoons butter, divided

½ cup minced onion

½ pound mushrooms, sliced

Salt and freshly ground pepper

3 pounds beef tenderloin, trimmed and cut into 1-inch by 2-inch pieces

1 cup low-sodium beef broth

⅛ teaspoon ground nutmeg

1 rounded teaspoon beef demi-glace*

1 tablespoon potato starch

1 cup low-fat sour cream

Cooked buttered gluten-free noodles, for serving

1. Heat the canola oil and 1 tablespoon of the butter over medium heat in a large, heavy skillet. Sauté the onions until golden brown and tender. Add the mushrooms and continue cooking until the mushrooms are tender and have released their juices. Set aside in a bowl. Season with the salt and pepper, to taste.

2. Season the beef with salt and pepper. Heat another tablespoon of the butter over high heat in the same skillet. Brown half the beef (about 3 minutes). The beef should be rosy inside; set aside in another bowl. Add the remaining butter to the skillet and repeat with the other half of the beef. Set aside in bowl.

3. Reduce the heat to medium. Deglaze the pan with the beef broth, Add the nutmeg and demi-glace. Stir to combine the demi-glace and cook until the liquid is reduced to ⅔ cup, about 3 to 4 minutes. Stir the potato starch into the sour cream and add to the skillet. Stir to combine into the sauce; simmer 2 minutes. Do not boil.

*We recommend More than Gourmet brand.

4. Add the mushrooms and any accumulated sauce back to the skillet; simmer for 1 minute. Add the beef and any accumulated sauce back to the skillet and stir to coat the beef with the sauce; simmer for 1 minute to rewarm. Add more salt and pepper, to taste. Serve immediately with buttered noodles.

BEEF STIR-FRY WITH OYSTER SAUCE

Stir-fries are the quintessential weeknight supper. Our beef with oyster sauce is flavorful, easy to make, and so delicious it could become habit forming. Serve it with brown rice and some quickly sautéed greens seasoned with a touch of sesame oil, and you've got an Asian-inspired meal you can throw together in less than 30 minutes at the end of a long day.

Serves 3–4

  1 pound flank steak or tenderloin, trimmed

  2 tablespoons canola oil

  2 teaspoons minced garlic

  2 teaspoons minced fresh ginger

  10 mushrooms, cleaned, trimmed, and sliced

  1 tablespoon low-sodium soy sauce

  3 tablespoons oyster sauce*

  1 tablespoon sesame oil

  ¼ cup scallions, thinly sliced

  Cooked rice, for serving

1. Thinly slice the meat on the diagonal into strips 1 inch wide and 2 inches long.

2. Heat the oil in a large, heavy skillet or wok over high heat. Add the garlic and cook until light brown.

3. Stir in the beef and ginger. Cook for 2 minutes, stirring constantly. Remove from the pan.

4. Add the mushrooms to the same skillet and sauté for 2 minutes.

5. Return the meat to the skillet and add the soy sauce and oyster sauce; cook for 1 minute. Remove from the heat and stir in the sesame oil and scallions. Serve warm over the rice.

* Gluten-free oyster sauce is available in natural food stores, specialty stores, and some grocery stores.

SOUTHWESTERN BRAISED CHUCK ROAST

We love the marriage of southwestern flavors with rich coffee and tomato, and our chuck roast showcases this matrimonial bliss in true style. Start this dish early in the afternoon so the whole house fills with delectable aromas. Serve it with mashed potatoes and plenty of fresh, steamed vegetables to soak up the thick sauce.

Serves 8

2 tablespoons olive oil

5 pounds chuck roast

Salt and freshly ground black pepper

1 tablespoon minced garlic

1 cup chopped onion

½ cup chopped celery

1 cup chopped red bell pepper

½ cup sliced carrot, cut into 2-inch pieces

1 small jalapeño pepper, seeded, finely chopped

½ cup red wine

1 tablespoon molasses

1 ancho chile, whole (or 1½ tablespoons ancho chile powder*)

2 teaspoons dried oregano

1 teaspoon ground cumin

1 cup strong freshly brewed coffee (not espresso or dark roast)

1 (14.5-ounce) can diced tomatoes (with juice)

1 tablespoon tomato paste

¼ cup chopped fresh cilantro, for sprinkling

1. Heat the oil in a large, heavy saucepan over medium-high heat. Sprinkle the chuck roast with the salt and pepper and add to the saucepan. Brown for 4 minutes per side. Transfer to a platter.

2. Add the garlic, onion, celery, red bell pepper, carrot, and jalapeño pepper to the saucepan. Reduce the heat to medium, cover, and cook until the onion is tender, stirring occasionally, about 5 minutes. Add the red wine and stir for 15 seconds. Add the

*Available in the spice section of most supermarkets and Latin markets.

molasses, ancho chile, oregano, cumin, coffee, tomatoes with juice, and tomato paste. Bring to a boil while scraping up the browned bits. Return the chuck and any juices to the pan and bring to a boil.

3. Cover, reduce the heat to low, and simmer until the meat is very tender, about 2 hours. Turn the chuck every 30 minutes while simmering. Season with more salt and pepper. Transfer the chuck to a platter.

4. Purée the sauce in a food processor (or with a hand processor) and then pour the sauce over the chuck. Sprinkle with the chopped cilantro and serve hot.

COOKS' NOTE:
Can be prepared 1 day ahead. Cool and cover with foil. Refrigerate until needed. Rewarm, covered in the oven, for 30 to 40 minutes at 350ºF.

BRISKET WITH BARBECUE SAUCE

What could be more effortless than throwing a brisket in the oven with some seasonings? Pulling it out several hours later and knowing that it will make a delicious dinner served with roasted vegetables, cole slaw, and corn bread. Try our brisket with its own savory barbecue sauce for a weekend dinner with family or friends. Enjoy the leftovers on Monday for another quick and easy meal.

Serves 6–8

1 tablespoon canola oil

1 4-pound flat-cut beef brisket, trimmed

1 (8-ounce) can tomato sauce

1 cup chopped onions

2 tablespoons molasses

1 tablespoon minced garlic

2 teaspoons ground cumin

2 teaspoons chili powder

Salt and freshly ground black pepper

COOKS' NOTES:
Sauce can be thickened, if desired. Combine about 2 rounded teaspoons of potato starch in a small bowl with about ½ cup of the sauce. Pour the thickened mixture into the remaining sauce and cook over medium-high heat until the sauce starts to thicken.

Brisket is best when made at least 1 day ahead and in fact can be made as many as 2 days ahead; store in a tightly sealed container in the refrigerator. Rewarm, covered, in the oven at 350ºF for 30 to 40 minutes, or until hot.

1. Place the rack in the center of the oven. Preheat the oven to 325ºF.

2. Heat the oil in a large, heavy (5-quart) Dutch oven or other large, covered, ovenproof pot over very high heat; brown the meat on both sides.

3. Combine the tomato sauce, chopped onions, molasses, garlic, cumin, and chili powder in a small bowl and pour it over the meat. Add the salt and pepper, to taste.

4. Cover the pot and place it in the oven. Cook for about 3 hours or until fork tender, turning once every hour.

5. Transfer the brisket to a plate or cutting board and allow it to cool for 1 hour. Trim any remaining fat and thinly slice across the grain. Return the meat to the pot and arrange the slices in the sauce in order to reheat. Rewarm, covered, in a preheated 350ºF oven and serve with the pan sauce.

GRILLED BEEF FILLET STEAKS WITH GARLIC PASTE

Cooking food over a fire is a time-honored way to bond with others. When it comes to summer grilling, we want steak, and we want it medium rare, please. This recipe is our favorite way to make grilled fillet; it never fails to make mouths water. Serve it with a big platter of colorful summer vegetables. Don't count on any leftovers.

Serves 10

> 5 pounds fillet of beef tenderloin, trimmed and cut into 2-inch-thick steaks
>
> ½ cup Newman's Own Olive Oil & Vinegar Dressing*
>
> 2 tablespoons finely minced garlic
>
> 3 tablespoons coarse sea salt
>
> 1 tablespoon coarsely cracked peppercorns

1. Place the steaks in a large, shallow dish. To make the marinade, combine the dressing and the garlic in a bowl. Spread 1 tablespoon of the marinade over each steak. Marinate overnight (or at least 2 hours) in the refrigerator.

2. Remove the steaks from the refrigerator and place the underside of each steak on top of another steak that is covered with the garlic paste. Move each steak around so it becomes slightly coated with the paste. Return each steak to the pan, underside facing up. Repeat until all steaks are coated on both sides.

3. Combine the salt and peppercorns in a small bowl. Sprinkle 1 teaspoon onto each steak and pat the mixture in. Bring the meat to room temperature. Preheat the grill to 450°F.

4. Grill the steaks for 5 minutes on each side (for medium rare). Serve hot.

---

* Although we like to use Newman's Own bottled dressings (they're of good quality and convenient), you can save money by making your own vinaigrette.

SAUTÉED PORK WITH MAPLE MUSTARD SAUCE

Pork with maple mustard sauce is an often-requested favorite in our homes. It pairs sweet maple syrup with spicy country mustard for a delectable pork dish you and your family will relish. Serve it with roasted cauliflower and sautéed spinach for a neutralizing dinner at the end of a long day.

Serves 4–6

1½ pounds pork tenderloin (or pork cutlets—if using cutlets, skip Steps 1 and 2)

Salt and freshly ground black pepper

1 teaspoon dried sage, divided

2 tablespoons butter, divided

⅔ cup low-sodium chicken broth

1 tablespoon pure maple syrup

1 tablespoon coarse-grained mustard

1. Trim the tenderloins and cut them into 1-inch-thick slices.

2. Place each pork slice between sheets of wax paper (or plastic wrap) and pound them to a ¼-inch thickness with a mallet or rolling pin.

3. Lay the pork slices on a plate and sprinkle with salt, pepper, and ¼ teaspoon of the sage. Turn them over and repeat, sprinkling with salt, pepper, and another ¼ teaspoon of the sage. Set aside. *Can be prepared up to 3 hours ahead. Cover tightly with plastic wrap and refrigerate.*

4. Melt 1 tablespoon of the butter in a large skillet over medium-high heat. Add half the pork slices and sauté for about 2 minutes per side, until browned and cooked through. Transfer to a plate and cover loosely with foil. Repeat with the remaining butter and pork slices. Transfer the cooked pork slices to the foil-covered plate.

5. Whisk together the broth, maple syrup, mustard, and remaining ½ teaspoon of the sage. Add the mixture to the skillet with the pan drippings. Scrape up the browned bits and boil until syrupy, about 2 minutes. Remove from the heat. Season to taste with more salt and pepper.

6. Return the pork slices to the heated sauce and turn them until each slice is coated. Serve immediately.

PORK WITH APPLES AND CALVADOS

Our Pork with Apples and Calvados is a wonderful fall meal. It combines fresh-picked apple flavor with savory herbs and tender pork. You can prep the pork ahead and then sauté it just before you serve the main course. Creamy mashed potatoes and a simple dish of roasted Brussels sprouts complete the autumn experience.

Serves 4–6

1½ pounds pork tenderloin (or pork cutlets—if using cutlets, skip Steps 1 and 2)

Salt and freshly ground black pepper

1½ teaspoons dried thyme, divided

¼ cup brown rice flour

3 medium Granny Smith apples

3 tablespoons unsalted butter, divided

2 teaspoons dark brown sugar

⅓ cup finely chopped shallots

2 tablespoons apple cider vinegar

¼ cup Calvados (or other apple brandy)

⅓ cup apple cider or juice (unfiltered is best)*

½ cup heavy cream

1. Trim the tenderloins and cut them into 1-inch-thick slices.

2. Place each pork slice between sheets of wax paper (or plastic wrap) and pound them to a ¼-inch thickness with a mallet or rolling pin.

3. Lay the pork slices on a plate and sprinkle with salt, pepper, and ½ teaspoon thyme. Lightly dredge the slices in the brown rice flour. Set aside. *Can be prepared up to 3 hours ahead. Cover tightly with plastic wrap and refrigerate.*

4. Peel, core, and slice each apple into 16 slices.

5. Melt 1 tablespoon of the butter in a large, heavy skillet on medium-high heat. Add the sugar and stir. Add the apples and sauté until golden brown and tender, about six minutes. Set aside in a microwaveable dish.

---

* If you have a professional stove top with extra-hot burners, you may need to add up to ½ cup apple cider.

6. In the same skillet, melt ½ tablespoon of the butter over medium-high heat. Add half the pork slices and sauté for about 2 minutes per side, until browned and cooked through. Transfer to a plate and cover loosely with foil. Repeat with another ½ tablespoon of the butter and the remaining pork slices. Transfer the cooked pork slices to the foil-covered plate.

7. Reduce the heat to low and melt the remaining tablespoon of butter in the same skillet. Add the remaining 1 teaspoon thyme and the shallots and sauté until the shallots are soft, about 2 minutes. Increase the heat to medium-high; add the apple cider vinegar and boil until syrupy. Turn off the heat and add the Calvados. Turn the heat back on to medium high and scrape up the browned bits. Boil until syrupy. Add the apple cider and heavy cream; boil until thickened to a saucelike consistency, about 2 to 3 minutes. Remove from the heat. Season with more salt and pepper, to taste.

8. Return the pork slices to the heated sauce and turn them until each slice is coated. Reheat the apple slices in the microwave. Serve the pork topped with the sauce and apple slices.

SLOW-BRAISED PULLED PORK

Melt-in-your-mouth tender and delicately spiced, our Slow-Braised Pulled Pork is one of those dishes our families eagerly anticipate. It should be started early on the day you plan to serve it—or better yet, the day before. No matter when you cook it, be prepared for the delicious aromas: members of your household will slyly circle the kitchen and make mad, kamikaze-style dives for the roast on the carving board. In our homes, boys, girls, and grown men have all sacrificed personal safety during repeated attempts to taste this succulent, flavorful roast while it was being cut up by a knife-wielding cook.

Our pulled pork recipe also provides a variety of delicious meal options. It can be served with our savory Red Bean Sauce (recipe follows), as a sandwich with barbecue sauce, or rolled into a corn tortilla. No matter how you serve it, you'll have a meal that's so tasty, your family members will regroup to plan their next raid on the leftovers.

Serves 8

> 1 tablespoon canola oil
>
> 1 (5½-pound) pork shoulder rump roast
>
> ½ cup low-sodium beef broth*
>
> 1 tablespoon tomato paste
>
> 1 tablespoon minced garlic
>
> 1 teaspoon ground cumin
>
> 1 teaspoon chili powder
>
> 1 teaspoon dried thyme
>
> 1 teaspoon sea salt
>
> 1 teaspoon freshly ground black pepper
>
> Red Bean Sauce (recipe follows), for serving

1. Place the rack in the center of the oven. Preheat the oven to 325°F.

2. Heat the oil in a large, heavy (5-quart) Dutch oven or other large, covered, ovenproof pot over very high heat; brown the meat on all sides.

3. Pour in the broth and add the tomato paste, garlic, cumin, chili powder, thyme, salt, and pepper.

---

* If you are using pork with no added enhancers or solutions, increase the broth amount to 2 cups (instead of ½ cup).

4. Cover the pot and place it in the oven. Baste and turn the meat every 45 minutes. Cook for 3 to 4 hours, or until the meat is fork tender and falling apart and the gravy is reduced. If the pot has a tight seal and the gravy isn't reducing, remove the lid for the last 1½ hours of cooking time.

5. Allow the meat to cool in the pot uncovered. Remove the meat and cut into chunks. Return the meat to the pot in order to reheat, or store in a tightly sealed container in the refrigerator. Rewarm, covered, in the oven for 30 to 40 minutes, or until hot, at 350ºF.

6. Serve with Red Bean Sauce (recipe follows), or with a favorite barbecue sauce.

Red Bean Sauce

2 teaspoons canola oil

1 dried ancho chili pepper

½ cup chopped onions

¼ cup finely chopped carrots

2 teaspoons minced garlic

1 (15.5-ounce) can red kidney beans, drained and rinsed

1 cup low-sodium chicken broth

2 teaspoons ground cumin

½ teaspoon salt

½ teaspoon coarsely ground black pepper

1. Heat the oil in a medium-sized, heavy saucepan over medium heat. Add the dried ancho chili pepper and cook for 1 minute, until softened. Add the onions, carrots, and garlic and cook until the onions are tender, about 5 minutes. Add the beans, chicken broth, cumin, salt, and pepper. Cover and simmer for 20 minutes. Remove and discard the ancho chili pepper.

2. Remove the bean mixture from the heat and purée in a blender. Reheat in a small saucepan or microwave as necessary; add more salt and pepper, to taste. Serve with the pork roast above.

COOKS' NOTE:
Can be made up to 2 days in advance. Cover and refrigerate until ready to use. May need to be thinned with additional broth.

GRILLED PORK TENDERLOIN TERIYAKI

Various versions of this simple recipe have been around for years—and here is ours. Soy sauce and a few pantry-ready seasonings combine to make fragrant, mouth-watering pork tenderloin with an Asian twist. Serve it with colorful grilled vegetables and sweet potatoes.

Serves 4–6

4 tablespoons soy sauce

2 tablespoons canola oil

1 tablespoon minced garlic

2 teaspoons dark brown sugar

1 teaspoon ground ginger

½ teaspoon freshly ground black pepper

1½ pounds (2 tenderloins, ¾ pound each) pork tenderloin, trimmed of any membranes

1. To make the marinade, combine the soy sauce, canola oil, garlic, brown sugar, ginger, and pepper in a bowl. Mix until smooth. Place the pork tenderloins in a large container, and pour the marinade over the pork tenderloins. Cover and refrigerate for a minimum of 3 hours or overnight.

2. Bring the meat to room temperature. Grease the grill racks with cooking spray. Preheat the barbecue to medium heat.

3. Grill the pork over medium heat (350ºF-400ºF) for 30 minutes, or until meat thermometer registers 155ºF. Turn the pork while cooking every 10 minutes and brush with the marinade. Transfer the pork to a cutting board and let rest for 10 minutes.

4. Carve the pork diagonally into thin slices and arrange on a serving platter. Serve immediately.

BABY-BACK RIBS
WITH SOUTHERN SPICE RUB

"Ribs for dinner!" Sounds good, doesn't it? Even better, it brings the family home and to the table in a hurry. Regrettably, many people don't think about making ribs unless they're having friends over for a barbecue. Others don't think about making ribs, period; they only eat ribs at restaurants. But once you try our special Southern Spice Rub (recipe follows) and our no-fuss method for cooking succulent and tender baby-back ribs, you'll wonder why you waited so long.

Serves 6–8

    2 slabs baby-back ribs (4–6 pounds total)

    ½ to 1 cup Southern Spice Rub (recipe follows)

    Barbecue sauce, for serving

1. Line a large roasting pan with a double layer of heavy-duty foil. Place the ribs in the pan, bone-side down, and sprinkle with ¼ to ½ cup of the Southern Spice Rub. Turn the ribs over, so the bone side is facing up, and sprinkle with an additional ¼ to ½ cup of the rub. Refrigerate for 30 minutes.

2. Bring the meat to room temperature. Preheat the oven to 325ºF. Cook for 60 minutes. Remove the pan from the oven and turn the ribs over. Return the pan to the oven and cook for another 60 minutes.

3. Increase the temperature to 350ºF. Remove the pan from the oven and lightly baste the ribs with your favorite barbecue sauce. Cover with foil. Return to the oven and continue to cook for 15 more minutes.

4. Turn off the oven and allow the ribs to sit in the warm oven for 30 to 60 minutes. Slice into individual portions and serve with your favorite barbecue sauce.

Southern Spice Rub

When using rubs, apply them to food that is completely dry. How much spice rub you use for each recipe is up to you, but a general rule is 3 tablespoons per 1 pound of food.

Yields 1¾ cups rub

¼ cup paprika

¼ cup cracked black pepper

¼ cup chili powder

¼ cup sea salt

¼ cup granulated sugar

2 tablespoons garlic powder

2 tablespoons onion powder

1 tablespoon dried thyme

½ teaspoon ground cayenne pepper, optional

COOKS' NOTE:
Leftover rub mixture can be stored for up to 1 year in a cool, dry place.

1. Combine paprika, black pepper, chili powder, salt, sugar, garlic powder, onion powder, thyme, and cayenne pepper (if using) in a medium-sized mixing bowl and whisk together. Transfer to an airtight container.

PORK TENDERLOIN WITH SOUTHERN SPICE RUB

We love to use our lip-smacking Southern Spice Rub on pork tenderloin. It is sure to please even the pickiest barbecue aficionados. Brush the tenderloins with your favorite barbecue sauce after you take them off the grill.

Serves 4–6

1½ pounds (2 tenderloins, ¾ pound each) pork tenderloin, trimmed of any membranes

4–5 tablespoons Southern Spice Rub (see page 246)

Barbecue sauce, for serving

1. Place the meat and the Southern Spice Rub into a large zip-top plastic bag and shake until the meat is evenly coated with the rub. Chill for 30 minutes.

2. Bring the meat to room temperature. Grease the grill racks with cooking spray and preheat the grill to medium heat.

3. Grill the pork over medium heat (350°F to 400°F) for 30 minutes, or until a meat thermometer registers 155°F. Turn the pork while cooking every 10 minutes to prevent the rub from burning. Transfer the pork to a cutting board and let stand for 10 minutes.

4. Carve the pork diagonally into thin slices and arrange on serving platter. Serve hot with your favorite barbecue sauce.

GRILLED PORK TENDERLOIN WITH ANCHO–CHIPOTLE CHILE MARINADE AND BLACK BEAN SAUCE

A blend of smoke, spice, and tangy flavors make this pork tenderloin sing. Serve it with mashed sweet potatoes and a multicolored platter of roasted vegetables for an out-of-the-ordinary meal you can enjoy with friends or family. For a delicious variation, make this same dish with beef tenderloin cut into 2-inch steaks (grill 5 minutes on each side for medium rare).

Serves 4–6

2 tablespoons canola oil

1 tablespoon honey

1 tablespoon red wine vinegar

2 tablespoons tomato sauce

½–1 teaspoon ancho chili powder*

½–1 teaspoon chipotle chili powder*

½ teaspoon salt

1½ pounds (2 tenderloins, ¾ pound each) pork tenderloin, trimmed of any membranes

Black Bean Sauce (recipe follows), for serving

1. To make the marinade, mix the oil, honey, vinegar, tomato sauce, ancho chili powder, chipotle chili powder, and salt in a small bowl. Place the pork in a flat dish and coat with the marinade. Cover with plastic wrap and refrigerate for 24 to 36 hours.

2. Allow the pork to come to room temperature. Grill over medium-high heat until the internal temperature registers 155°F. Allow pork to rest for 10 minutes before slicing. Serve with Black Bean Sauce (recipe follows).

* Available in the spice section of most supermarkets and Latin markets.

Black Bean Sauce

1 tablespoon canola oil

1 cup chopped onions

⅓ cup finely chopped carrot

1 medium-sized jalapeño pepper, seeded and minced

1 tablespoon minced garlic

2 (15.5-ounce) cans black beans, drained and rinsed

2 cups low-sodium chicken broth

2 teaspoons ground cumin

½ teaspoon salt

½ teaspoon coarsely ground black pepper

1. Heat the oil in a medium-sized, heavy saucepan over medium heat. Add the onions, carrot, jalapeño pepper, and garlic and cook until the onions are tender, about 5 minutes. Add the beans, chicken broth, cumin, salt, and pepper. Cover and simmer for 30 minutes.

2. Remove the bean mixture from the heat and purée it in a blender. Reheat the purée in a small saucepan; add more salt and pepper, to taste. Serve with the Grilled Pork Tenderloin with Ancho–Chipotle Chile Marinade.

COOKS' NOTE:
Can be made up to 2 days in advance. Cover and refrigerate until ready to use. May need to be thinned with additional broth.

ROASTED LEG OF LAMB WITH GARLIC CRUST

Lamb is the "middle child" of the American meat family: it delivers the goods, but it is so underappreciated. This recipe is lamb's coming-out party. We love to serve it with a creamy potato gratin and a simple green vegetable, like roasted asparagus. Pour a glass of hearty red wine and enjoy a delectable, aromatic meal.

Serves 6–8

1 (5–6 pound) leg of lamb (allow 1 pound per person of uncooked trimmed leg of lamb)

Olive oil

¼ cup minced garlic

Dried rosemary

Salt and freshly ground black pepper

1. Place the lamb on a roasting rack in a shallow roasting pan. Trim the excess fat and make 10 to 12 long, shallow slits in the meat. Rub the entire leg with olive oil. Spread the crushed garlic over the top and sides of the meat, pushing gently into the slits. Sprinkle the meat liberally with the rosemary, salt, and pepper. Allow the lamb to come to room temperature.

2. Preheat the oven to 425°F. Place the rack in the center of the oven.

3. Place the pan on the oven rack just below the center of the oven and roast for 15 minutes; turn the oven heat down to 350°F. Roast for another hour, until the internal temperature registers 145°F for medium rare, or 155°F for medium. Allow to rest for 15 minutes before carving.

MOROCCAN LAMB STEW

This incredible dish blends the subtle flavors of northern Africa into a fragrant and substantial stew that is as beautiful to look at as it is to eat. At first glance, this recipe looks difficult, but it really a one-dish main course of vibrant colors and rich textures that can be ready in 1 hour. It's perfect for a dinner party. (See Cooks' Insight on the following page and our Moroccan Chicken Stew variation below.)

Serves 6

¼ cup olive oil, divided

2 pounds boneless lamb, cut into 2-inch chunks

1 cup thinly sliced onion

1 tablespoon minced garlic

1 tablespoon minced peeled ginger

1 tablespoon paprika

1 teaspoon ground turmeric

½ teaspoon ground coriander

½ teaspoon ground cumin

¼ teaspoon cayenne pepper

¼ teaspoon ground cinnamon

¼ teaspoon crumbled saffron

2 cups low-sodium beef broth

1 cup canned diced tomatoes in juice

1 cup drained canned garbanzo beans (chickpeas)

½ teaspoon freshly ground black pepper

1 teaspoon salt

1 cup red bell pepper, cored seeded and cut into strips 1 inch thick by 2 inches long

1 cup carrots or fresh pumpkin, peeled and strips 1 inch thick by 2 inches long

1 cup zucchini, cut into strips 1 inch thick by 2 inches long

1 cup green beans, cut into 2-inch strips

½ cup golden raisins

¼ cup chopped fresh cilantro

4 cups freshly cooked brown rice, for serving

1 lemon, thinly sliced, for garnish

Fresh mint, for garnish

1. Heat 2 tablespoons of the olive oil in a large, heavy pot and lightly brown the lamb in batches over medium-high heat. Remove the lamb to a large bowl and set aside.

2. Heat the remaining 2 tablespoons of the olive oil in the same pot over medium-high heat. Add the onion, garlic, and ginger and sauté until the onion is translucent, about 10 minutes. Add the paprika, turmeric, coriander, cumin, cayenne, and cinnamon and stir for 1 minute.

3. Add the saffron, broth, tomatoes, garbanzo beans, salt, and pepper and bring to a boil. Reduce the heat and simmer, covered, for 10 minutes.

4. Add the lamb and return to a boil. Reduce the heat, cover, and simmer for 30 minutes.

5. Add the red pepper and carrots and cook for 10 minutes. Stir in the zucchini, green beans, raisins, and cilantro and simmer, covered, until the vegetables are tender, about 5 minutes.

6. Season with more salt and pepper, to taste. Serve the hot stew over the rice. Garnish with fresh lemon slices and mint.

Moroccan Chicken Stew Variation

• Replace lamb with 4 boneless chicken breasts, skin removed, each cut into 2-inch pieces, and 4 boneless chicken thighs, skin removed, each cut into 2-inch pieces. Replace low-sodium beef broth with low-sodium chicken broth. Follow the directions for Steps 1–3. Add the chicken and return to a boil. Reduce the heat and simmer, covered, for 15 minutes. Follow the directions for Steps 5 and 6.

GRILLED TANDOORI LAMB WITH CUCUMBER RAITA

Even if you don't have a clay tandoor oven, you can make delicious tandoori-style lamb. All you need is a well stocked pantry of spices and some whole-milk yogurt. Everyone will relish the warm Indian flavors that enhance this succulent lamb dish. Serve it with grilled potatoes, okra, and Cucumber Raita (recipe follows).

Serves 4–8

- 2 cups plain whole-milk yogurt, divided
- 2 tablespoons fresh lemon juice
- 2 tablespoons peeled and minced fresh ginger
- 1 tablespoon minced garlic
- 1 teaspoon salt
- 1 teaspoon ground coriander
- 1 teaspoon ground turmeric
- ½ teaspoon saffron threads, crumbled
- ½ teaspoon ground cumin
- ½ teaspoon freshly ground black pepper
- ½ teaspoon cayenne pepper
- 2 pounds boneless loin of lamb, cut into 2-inch cubes
- 2 tablespoons olive oil
- ¼ cup chopped fresh cilantro, for sprinkling

1. To make the marinade, blend 1 cup of the yogurt with the lemon juice, ginger, garlic, salt, coriander, turmeric, saffron threads, cumin, black pepper, and cayenne pepper and process in a food processor until smooth. Transfer to a large bowl and mix in the remaining cup of yogurt.

2. Add the lamb cubes to the marinade; turn to coat. Cover and refrigerate overnight.

3. Preheat the grill to 400°F. Divide the lamb evenly among 8 long metal skewers. Grill for 10 minutes, turning and basting evenly with the marinade.

4. To finish, baste 1 side of the lamb with the olive oil; cook for 2 minutes. Turn, baste the other side of the lamb with the oil, and cook another 2 minutes.

5. Transfer to a platter, sprinkle with the cilantro, and serve hot.

Grilled Tandoori Chicken Variation

• Replace the lamb with 8 skinless chicken thigh pieces. Grill the chicken for 15 minutes, turning every 5 minutes and basting evenly with the marinade. Proceed with Steps 4–5 in the main recipe.

Cucumber Raita

> 1 cup plain yogurt
>
> ¼ cup cucumber, peeled, seeded, and cut into small cubes
>
> 1 teaspoon chopped fresh mint leaves
>
> ½ teaspoon ground cumin
>
> ½ teaspoon salt
>
> Freshly ground black pepper
>
> ⅛ teaspoon cayenne pepper

1. Pour the yogurt into a small mixing bowl and beat with a fork until smooth. Add the cucumber, mint, cumin, salt, black pepper, and cayenne pepper. Mix well and serve chilled.

BUFFALO MEATBALLS

Enjoy the delicious benefits of eating all-natural buffalo meat in this very traditional dish. Hearty and filled with the earthy flavors of Parmesan and Italian herbs, this dish is so good that you may never reach for regular ground chuck again.

12 meatballs

> 1 pound fresh ground buffalo meat
>
> ¼ cup gluten-free bread crumbs*
>
> ¼ cup grated Parmesan cheese
>
> 1 large egg
>
> 1 tablespoon minced fresh garlic
>
> 1 teaspoon oregano
>
> ½ teaspoon basil
>
> ½ teaspoon freshly ground black pepper
>
> ¼ teaspoon salt
>
> 3 cups prepared pasta sauce of choice
>
> Cooked gluten-free pasta or gluten-free bread, for serving

1. Preheat the oven to 400°F. Place the rack in the bottom third of the oven. Lightly grease a rimmed baking sheet.

2. In a medium-sized mixing bowl, combine the buffalo meat with the bread crumbs, Parmesan cheese, egg, garlic, oregano, basil, pepper, and salt. Mix until just blended.

3. Form 12 meatballs and space them evenly on the rimmed baking sheet. Bake at 400°F for 15 minutes. Remove the baking sheet from the oven and transfer the meatballs to a large, heavy saucepan. Add the pasta sauce, cover the pan, and simmer for 30 to 60 minutes. Serve hot with your favorite gluten-free pasta or as a meatball sub on gluten-free bread.

* An economical, easy to make gluten-free bread crumb recipe is available in *Gluten-Free Baking Classics, Second Edition*, by Annalise Roberts (Surrey Books, 2008). You can also simply grind up the ends of a loaf of gluten-free bread in a blender or food processor and then bake the crumbs in the oven at 325°F until lightly browned.

VEAL MEATBALL STROGANOFF

Reminiscent of Swedish meatballs, this kid-pleasing favorite is one of the most requested meals we make in our homes. It is comfort food at its best—tender meatballs in a creamy sour cream-based sauce, served over buttered noodles. Toss a green salad, steam some broccoli, and you've got a great dinner everyone in your home can enjoy.

Serves 4–6

Meatballs

1½ pounds ground veal

¾ cups fresh gluten-free bread crumbs*

1 large egg

2 tablespoons milk

½ teaspoon dried thyme

⅛ teaspoon black pepper

¼ teaspoon salt

Sauce

1 tablespoon canola oil

¾ cup minced onions

1½ cups low-sodium chicken broth

½ teaspoon thyme

1 heaping teaspoon veal or chicken demi-glace**

1 tablespoon potato starch

1 cup low-fat sour cream

Salt and freshly ground black pepper

Gluten-free buttered noodles, for serving

1. Preheat the oven to 425°F. Place the rack in the bottom third of the oven. Lightly grease a rimmed baking sheet.

* An economical, easy to make gluten-free bread crumb recipe is available in *Gluten-Free Baking Classics, Second Edition*, by Annalise Roberts (Surrey Books, 2008). You can also simply grind up the ends of a loaf of gluten-free bread in a blender or food processor and then bake the crumbs in the oven at 325°F until lightly browned.
** We recommend More than Gourmet brand.

2. To make the meatballs, combine the veal, bread crumbs, egg, milk, thyme, pepper, and salt in the large bowl of an electric mixer. Mix at medium speed until just blended. (Do not overmix.)

3. Form 16 meatballs and space them evenly on the rimmed baking sheet. Bake at 400°F for 15 minutes.

4. Make the sauce while the meatballs are baking. Heat the oil over medium heat in a large, heavy skillet. Sauté the onions until golden brown and tender. Add the chicken broth, thyme, and demi-glace. Stir to combine and cook over low heat for 2 minutes.

5. Add the cooked meatballs to the sauce. Cover the skillet and simmer over very low heat for 20 minutes. Stir the potato starch into the sour cream and add the mixture to the skillet; stir to combine. Add the salt and pepper, to taste. Cover and simmer another 2 to 3 minutes, until heated through. Serve with gluten-free buttered noodles.

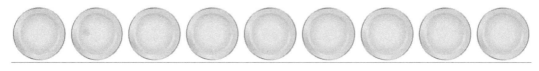

CHAPTER 12

Desserts

This section is not your typical dessert chapter. Our baking bible is Annalise's *Gluten-Free Baking Classics*, and we highly recommend it for your baking needs, including muffins, cakes, pies, cookies, and breads. We believe desserts should be a delicious treat, not an everyday rite of passage. Desserts shouldn't contain dried kale or some other decidedly nondessert ingredient, nor should they be considered healthy just because they include a ¼ cup of whole-grain flour. Thinking like that only clouds the distinction between where the meal ends and dessert begins.

For the most part, desserts *aren't* healthy: they contain a lot of sugar and some sort of fat, and they don't help build your immune system. But we love them anyway. Therefore, we offer a small collection of desserts that we like to make for our own families. Each of these recipes feature some sort of whole food, such as fresh fruit, tofu, pumpkin, or Neufchâtel cream cheese (okay, maybe cream cheese is a stretch, but it's a kid favorite).

Strawberries Drizzled with Chocolate

Caramelized Grilled Pineapple

Rhubarb Strawberry Fool

Poached Seasonal Fruits

Cold Lemon Soufflé

Pumpkin Pie Pudding

Caramel Cheesecake Pie

Rich Chocolate Mousse

STRAWBERRIES DRIZZLED WITH CHOCOLATE

This recipe is elegant simplicity at its best. Kids of all ages seem to love this easy-to-make treat. Why spend time dipping individual strawberries when you can create an enticing platter of self-indulgent goodness in less than 5 minutes. Try our chocolate-covered strawberries with your family or friends and you'll see why we make it all the time.

Makes 1 large platter

4 cups fresh strawberries, with green tops removed

12 ounces semisweet, bittersweet, or white chocolate, coarsely chopped

Mint leaves, for garnish

1. Arrange the berries on a serving platter. Stir the chocolate in the top of a double boiler set over simmering water until completely melted and smooth. (See the Cooks' Note at right for instructions for melting the chocolate in a microwave.) Remove the chocolate from over the water. Drizzle the melted chocolate decoratively over the strawberries. If using both semisweet or bittersweet chocolate and white chocolate, alternate lines for a beautiful presentation.

2. Chill until the chocolate is set, about 30 minutes and up to 6 hours. Garnish with fresh mint leaves and serve.

COOKS' NOTE:
Alternatively, the chocolate can be melted in the microwave. To do so, place the chocolate in a glass bowl and microwave on medium-high for 90 seconds, removing the mixture from the microwave every 30 seconds to stir it with a rubber spatula as it melts. Once it is smooth, drizzle the chocolate over the berries.

CARAMELIZED GRILLED PINEAPPLE

This is an incredibly delicious dessert you can make in minutes. It's the perfect way to bring any dinner to a sweet end.

Serves 4

1 large whole pineapple

2 tablespoons unsalted butter

2 tablespoons packed brown sugar (preferably dark)

2 tablespoons rum (preferably dark)

Ice cream, for serving (optional)

1. Preheat the grill to 425°F.

2. Trim the pineapple leaves to about 2 inches. Quarter the pineapple lengthwise. Cut and discard the cores from the quarters. With a sharp knife, cut the fruit from the rinds, keeping the rinds intact and reserving them. Cut the pineapple crosswise into ½-inch-thick slices.

3. In a small saucepan, cook the butter, brown sugar, and rum over moderate heat, stirring constantly, for 1 minute. Add the pineapple, stirring until coated, and cook mixture for 1 minute more. Remove the pineapple from the saucepan and place the pieces on a platter.

4. Transfer the pineapple to the grill. Grill the pineapple for 3 to 4 minutes on each side, or until slightly charred and heated through.

5. Arrange the grilled pineapple evenly into the four pineapple rinds. Serve the pineapple with the ice cream, if desired.

RHUBARB STRAWBERRY FOOL

One of the first vegetables to hit the markets each spring, rhubarb has been used since ancient times as a traditional Chinese medicine to balance and purify the gastrointestinal tract. This underappreciated vegetable is nobody's fool. We begin making this light creamy dessert in April—not only to celebrate the arrival of spring, but also to add a nutritional boost to any meal.

Makes 2 cups

> 2 cups rhubarb (about 2 large stalks), diced into 1-inch pieces*
>
> ⅓ cup granulated sugar
>
> 1 teaspoon finely chopped crystallized ginger
>
> 1 teaspoon finely grated orange zest
>
> ¼ cup fresh orange juice
>
> 1 cup strawberries hulled and cut into halves (or use whole raspberries)
>
> 8 ounces silken tofu

1. Combine the rhubarb, sugar, ginger, orange zest, and orange juice in a medium-size, heavy saucepan. Stir well and bring to a boil over medium heat. Reduce the heat, cover loosely, and simmer for 4 minutes.

2. Add the strawberries and cook for 1 minute longer. Remove from the heat and cool to room temperature.

3. In a food processor, puree the silken tofu until smooth. Add in the cooked, cooled compote and blend until smooth. Cool in the refrigerator. Serve cold.

COOKS' NOTE:
The compote can be made several days ahead and refrigerated.

* Rhubarb leaves are inedible. Trim the stalks thoroughly before cooking.

POACHED SEASONAL FRUITS

Whenever we serve this classic and elegant dessert, it always gets rave reviews. Poached fruit is a colorful celebration of seasonal sweetness, and we wouldn't have it any other way—except to eat it more often.

Serves 4

1 cup water

1 cup sweet white wine

½ cup granulated sugar

1 vanilla bean, split

8 fresh apricots, small peaches, or nectarines, halved, pits removed

2 tablespoons Grand Marnier liqueur or brandy

1 tablespoon chopped crystallized ginger

2 gluten-free gingersnap cookies, crumbled

2 cups vanilla yogurt, for serving

1. To make the syrup, combine the water, wine, sugar, and vanilla bean in a large skillet over medium-high heat. Bring to a boil, reduce the heat to medium-low, and then stir at a simmer until the sugar has dissolved, about 5 minutes.

2. Add the apricots, pit-side down, and allow the syrup to return to a simmer. Then reduce the heat further to a very gentle simmer. Cook for 4 minutes and then carefully turn the fruit over. Cook for 1 more minute, or until the fruit is tender. Remove the apricots with a slotted spoon to a serving dish. Set aside.

3. Boil the syrup for 5 minutes, until thick. Cool for 2 minutes and then add the Grand Marnier. Pour the syrup over the apricots.

4. Sprinkle the apricots with the ginger and crumbled cookies. Serve with the vanilla yogurt (and of course, more cookies).

Variation

- Instead of apricots, use 12 fresh plums, halved, pits removed. Replace the syrup ingredients listed in Step 1 with the following: 1½ cups water; 1 cup Port wine; ½ cup sugar; ½ vanilla bean, split; 2 cardamom pods; and 2 tablespoons brandy. Prepare according to the same method.

COLD LEMON SOUFFLÉ

If you've been yearning to add a little tofu to your diet and you want to start with something easy and delicious, search no more. Our cold lemon soufflé has a creamy texture and rich lemon flavor that belies an interesting detail: it uses silken tofu instead of 1 cup of heavy cream. We've lightened up one of our favorite desserts with nutritious soy, but no one will know unless you tell. The result is a light, tangy dessert with less fat, calories, and guilt. We think it's the perfect way to end a meal. Enjoy a dish of this luscious treat with a ginger cookie.

Serves 8

> 2 packages unflavored gelatin
> ½ cup water
> 1 cup silken tofu, drained
> ½ cup heavy cream
> 6 fresh large egg yolks
> 1½ cups granulated sugar
> 1 tablespoon grated lemon rind
> ⅔ cup fresh lemon juice
> Lemon slices, for garnish
> Mint leaves, for garnish

1. Combine the gelatin with the water in a small saucepan. Let stand for 10 minutes to soften. Stir over low heat until the gelatin is dissolved; remove and cool slightly.

2. Blend the tofu in a food processor until smooth. Set aside.

3. Beat the heavy cream in the large bowl of an electric mixer until very light and thick; refrigerate until needed.

4. Beat the egg yolks and sugar in the large bowl of an electric mixer with clean beaters at high speed until very light and thick.

5. Stir the lemon rind and juice into the gelatin. Pour the lemon–gelatin mixture into the egg mixture. Add the silken tofu and beat at a low speed until blended.

6. Chill the lemon mixture in the refrigerator, stirring occasionally, until it mounds softly with a spoon (it should not be stiff). This step takes approximately 20 minutes.

7. Fold the chilled lemon mixture into the whipped cream until there are no white stripes; pour the mixture into a soufflé dish. Chill for several hours before serving.

8. Garnish with the thin lemon slices and fresh mint leaves.

PUMPKIN PIE PUDDING

We gobble up this easy-to-make, high-fiber pudding all fall and winter long, and our bodies thank us for it. Between the soy (rich in high-quality protein, calcium, and iron), the pumpkin (rich in Vitamin E, beta carotene, and potassium), and the anti-inflammatory benefits of the cinnamon, it's hard to say no to a second helping. For a more savory version, cut the brown sugar to half a cup and serve with yogurt and nuts.

Serves 8

12 ounces silken tofu

2 cups canned pumpkin

¾ cup dark brown sugar

1 teaspoon ground cinnamon

½ teaspoon ground ginger

¼ teaspoon ground cloves

¼ teaspoon ground nutmeg

1. Preheat the oven to 350°F. Place the rack in the center of the oven. Lightly grease an 8-inch soufflé dish or pie pan with cooking spray.

2. In a blender or food processor, purée together the tofu and pumpkin until smooth. Add the brown sugar, cinnamon, ginger, cloves, and nutmeg and blend thoroughly.

3. Pour the mixture into the pie dish and bake for 40 to 45 minutes, until set. Cool to room temperature before serving.

CARAMEL CHEESECAKE PIE*

When a whole cheesecake seems like too much, this pie is the perfect solution. The smooth caramel topping and creamy filling makes it one of the most requested desserts in our homes. Plan to serve it Sunday night and you won't have to worry about who will be home for dinner.

Makes 1 8-inch pie

Crust

1 cup Brown Rice Flour Mix (see the Baking Appendix F, page 286)

¼ cup ground hazelnuts or walnuts

1 teaspoon xanthan gum

5 tablespoons unsalted butter, room temperature.

¼ cup granulated sugar

1 large egg yolk

Grated rind of 1 lemon, optional

Cake Filling

20 ounces Neufchâtel cream cheese at room temperature

¾ cup granulated sugar

1½ tablespoons Brown Rice Flour Mix (see the Baking Appendix F, page 286)

⅛ teaspoon salt

3 large eggs

1 tablespoon heavy cream

1 tablespoon grated orange rind

Caramel Sauce

⅔ cup dark brown sugar

¼ cup (½ stick) unsalted butter

¼ cup heavy cream

1. Preheat the oven to 400ºF. Position the rack in the center of the oven. Spray a deep dish 8-inch pie pan with cooking spray. Generously dust with rice flour.

2. To make the crust, mix the Brown Rice Flour Mix, nuts, xanthan gum, butter, sugar, egg yolk, and lemon rind in the bowl of an electric mixer at low speed. Press the dough into the pie pan and bake for 12 minutes, until very light golden. Remove from the oven and cool slightly on a wire rack. Raise the oven temperature to 425ºF.

Note: This pie should be prepared at least 4 hours before serving.

3. To make the cake filling, beat the cream cheese until smooth in the large bowl of an electric mixer at medium speed. Reduce the speed and slowly add the sugar, Brown Rice Flour Mix, salt, eggs, cream, and orange rind. Scrape the bowl and beat at high speed for 5 minutes.

4. Pour the cream cheese mixture into the cooled pie crust. Bake in the center of the oven for 10 minutes. Reduce the oven temperature to 300°F and bake for 30 minutes more. Remove from the oven and cool on a wire rack while preparing the caramel sauce.

5. To make the caramel sauce, whisk together the brown sugar and butter in a heavy saucepan over medium-high heat until the butter melts. Whisk in the cream and stir until the sugar dissolves and the sauce is smooth, about 3 minutes. Pour the sauce evenly over the cooled pie and bring to room temperature. Chill the pie for at least 4 hours prior to serving.

RICH CHOCOLATE MOUSSE

We love this mousse recipe because it's as healthy as it's going to get without sacrificing flavor and texture. It's also wonderful because it has reduced calories and increased versatility. Serve it alone with fresh berries, or as a scooped topping for a flourless chocolate or angel-food cake. During the holidays, serve it piped into molded chocolate cups topped with crushed candy canes. It's always a crowd pleaser.

Serves 8

12 ounces silken tofu, drained

8 ounces dark chocolate, chopped

1 teaspoon pure vanilla extract

3 large egg whites

¼ teaspoon salt

½ cup granulated sugar

1. Blend the tofu in a food processor until smooth. Set aside.

2. Melt the chocolate in a heavy saucepan, stirring frequently to prevent burning. (See the Cooks' Note at right for instructions for melting the chocolate in a microwave.)

3. Add the melted chocolate to the tofu and blend until creamy. Add the vanilla and set aside.

4. Combine the egg whites and salt in the large bowl of an electric mixer. Start the mixer at medium speed and beat until the whites are foamy. Gradually increase the speed to high. Add the sugar 2 tablespoons at a time, beating until the sugar dissolves and the whites form stiff peaks. Do not scrape the bowl while beating.

5. Stir 1 cup of the beaten egg whites into the chocolate mixture and blend. Then fold in the remaining egg whites until it is thoroughly mixed.

6. Pour the mousse into serving bowls and chill in the refrigerator for at least 4 hours.

COOKS' NOTES:
You can also spoon the mousse into pre-made individual pastry or meringue shells or chocolate cups.

Alternatively, the chocolate can be melted in the microwave. To do so, place the chocolate in a glass bowl and microwave on medium-high for 90 seconds, removing the mixture from the microwave every 30 seconds to stir it with a rubber spatula as it melts. Once it is smooth, drizzle the chocolate over the berries.

Why Is Wheat Unhealthy?

REFINED WHITE FLOUR has rightfully been condemned for its lack of nutritional value and high glycemic index, but whole grains have long been praised as a good natural source of nutrition and fiber. The notion that wheat is unhealthy is definitely not the norm, but in light of the massive popularity of the Atkins and South Beach Diets, more and more people are beginning to view wheat with skepticism. Wheat, whether it's refined or whole, contributes to excess acidity in our bodies, and nutritionally speaking, it's hardly the powerhouse food it is marketed as, particularly when you compare it to other whole foods:

- Fresh vegetables and fruit, seafood, and lean meats all deliver more vitamins, minerals, and phytochemicals on a per-calorie basis than whole wheat.
- Fresh vegetables and fruits, nuts, and seeds deliver more fiber per serving than whole wheat.

To make matters worse, most breads that are labeled as "whole grain" contain refined whole wheat, which can spike your body's insulin levels and cause it to store excess energy as fat.

But the number one reason why wheat is unhealthy for many of us is that it contains gluten, a protein molecule that causes inflammation and chronic disease in the bodies of people who are sensitive to it. The only way to avoid eating gluten is to eat a diet that's free of wheat, rye, and barley. Research has shown that gluten-free diets not only reduce cardiovascular risk factors, including high cholesterol, but they also decrease the incidence of arthritis,[1] type-1 diabetes,[2] thyroid disease, lupus, and other autoimmune diseases.[3] In addition, there is evidence that autistic children who have been put on a gluten- and dairy-free diet show improvement in a variety of symptoms.[4]

APPENDIX A REFERENCES

1. Elkan, A., Sjoberg, B., Kolsrud, B., Hafstrom, B., and Frostegard, J. 2008. "The Gluten-Free Vegan Diet Induces Decreased LDL and Oxidized LDL Levels and Raised Atheroprotective Natural Antibodies against Phosphorylcholine in Patients with Rheumatoid Arthritis: A Randomized Study." *Arthritis Research Therapy* 10(2): R34.

2. Frisk, G., T. Hansson, I. Dahlbom, and T. Tuvemo. 2008. "A Unifying Hypothesis on the Development Of Type 1 Diabetes and Celiac Disease: Gluten Consumption May Be a Shared Causative Factor." Uppsala, Sweden: Department of Women's and Children's Health, Uppsala University, Akademiska Hospital. Medical Hypothesis 70(6): 1207-9.

3. Treem, W. 2004. "Emerging Concepts in Celiac Disease." *Current Opinion in Pediatrics* 16:552–9.

4. Reichelt, K., J. Ekrem, and H. Scott. 1990. "Gluten, Milk Proteins and Autism: Dietary Intervention Effects on Behavior and Peptide Section." *Journal of Applied Nutrition* 42:1–11.

Food Sensitivity—Food Allergies versus Food Intolerances

FOOD SENSITIVITY is the general term used to refer to individualistic adverse reactions to food or food components (usually proteins). Reactions that involve the immune system are called food allergies, and those that may or may not involve the immune system are called food intolerances.

A food allergy is an immediate hypersensitive immunologic response to a food protein and involves the immediate formation of allergen-specific immunoglobulin E (IgE) antibodies, with symptoms occurring shortly after eating the offending food. For example, a peanut allergy is an immediate immunologic response to the peanut protein. True food allergies are only a fraction of all food sensitivities.[1] It is estimated that as many as 12 million Americans have food allergies of one type or another. Approximately 90 percent of all IgE-mediated food allergies are caused by the "Big Eight" food sources of allergens: peanuts, tree nuts, milk, eggs, soybeans, fish, crustacean (shellfish), and wheat.

Food intolerance is a delayed hypersensitivity and can be caused by the absence of specific chemicals or enzymes needed to digest a food substance, or to the body's responses to certain food components both natural and artificial. For example, lactose intolerance is caused by the body's inability to produce enough lactase to break down the lactose present in milk.

Symptoms of food sensitivity vary greatly, and it can be hard to determine at what level of the spectrum a reaction is occurring. While true allergies are associated with fast-acting IgE responses (requiring the participation of antibodies), it can be difficult to determine which specific food causes other sensitivity because if the immune system is involved, the response is likely to be immunoglobulin G (IgG) mediated (a cellular reaction that requires the participation of T-lymphocytes, a type of white blood cell that helps the body fight infection) and to take place over a prolonged period of time. Thus, the causative agent and the response are separated in time, and may not be obviously related.

THE GLUTEN SENSITIVITY SPECTRUM

Gluten, a protein molecule with a unique sequence and structure, is found in wheat, barley, and rye, but not in oats, corn, or rice.[2] Gluten sensitivity enteropathy (enteropathy means any disease of the intestine) is associated with a variety of symptoms and health conditions. Gluten sensitivity includes wheat and gluten allergies, wheat intolerance, and gluten intolerance. There are two types of gluten intolerance, nonceliac and celiac disease.

Celiac Disease

Celiac disease is a genetic autoimmune disease that results from an inability to tolerate gluten. When people with celiac disease consume gluten, their body launches an immune attack on the lining of the small intestine. The small intestine is lined with tiny fingerlike projections called villi, which secrete digestive enzymes and absorb nutrients. With celiac disease, the villi are damaged or destroyed, resulting in the poor absorption of nutrients.

Celiac disease is the most prevalent chronic autoimmune disease, and because it is genetic, it runs in families. It can manifest itself anytime during a person's life and often becomes active for the first time after a time of stress, pregnancy, surgery, or a viral infection. One percent of all Americans are estimated to have celiac disease. The disease is recognized worldwide in countries populated by persons of European, Asian, Middle East, South American, and North African ancestry.[3] Following are some statistics on the prevalence of celiac disease in the United States:[4]

Prevalence of Celiac Disease in the United States[8]
Among healthy people: 1 in 100
Among people with related symptoms: 1 in 56
Among people with first-degree relatives (a parent, child, or sibling) who are celiac: 1 in 22
Among people with second-degree relatives (an aunt, uncle, or cousin) who are celiac: 1 in 39

More than 200 symptoms are associated with celiac disease, and almost everyone has a different set of symptoms. The most common symptoms include diarrhea, gas, bloating, vomiting, constipation, nausea, skin irritation, anemia, weight loss, chronic fatigue, weakness, joint pain, muscle cramps, neurologic complaints, migraine headaches, body aches, thyroid problems, and concentration and memory problems. Malabsorption caused by celiac disease can have serious side effects on many other organs of the body and can lead to other autoimmune diseases, cancer, diabetes, and heart disease.[5]

A person has to have specific genes in order to develop celiac disease. The two specific genes that have been recognized so far are part of the HLA Class II DQ genes, HLA-DQ2 and

HLA-DQ8. HLA are human leukocyte protein antigens, which are found on the surface of almost every cell in the body. The HLAs patrol the immune system and identify other cells as self (belonging to the body) or nonself (a foreign substance). They are thought to play a role in the development of certain genetically predisposed diseases, such as diabetes and celiac disease. This is because the genes that predispose people to autoimmune diseases may also control HLAs.[6]

The HLA is not just a genetic fingerprint. There is a reason why people with a particular HLA develop the disease. The enterocytes, the cells on the lining of the small intestine, have some receptors that are programmed by the Class II antigens to recognize and react to gluten (remember, an antigen is any substance that causes your immune system to produce antibodies against it). When people with celiac disease eat gluten, the gluten is attracted to and binds to HLA receptors that are present on all the cells that line their small intestine. In other words, the gluten nonself attaches to the body self, thereby creating a kind of receptor-gluten complex that is recognized by the body as nonself.

The HLA receptors then act as gatekeeper escorts and permit the gluten to enter the intestinal cell membrane and pass through into the mucosa lining of the small intestine. From the mucosa, this receptor-gluten complex enters the bloodstream and is responsible for producing toxic compounds that are ultimately responsible for tissue damage in the intestine. To complicate matters, people with celiac disease have certain antibodies that, because of genetics, are preprogrammed to look like the receptor-gluten complex. The white blood T-cells are not able to discriminate between the original receptor-gluten complexes and the antibodies that mimic them, although it remains a mystery why certain antibodies mimic gluten proteins.[7]

The body's white blood T-cells then release messages to the white blood B-cells to create antibodies against the receptor-gluten complex and the antibodies that mimic them and attack. This action triggers an autoimmune attack that causes other immune system T-cells to destroy the intestinal villi; the body is literally attacking itself. Depending on the person, this immune response can also create inflammation in other parts of the body.

The diagnostic criteria for celiac disease are very clear and specific. Initial screening is done by blood tests, including tissue transglutaminase TTG-IgA/IgG and endomysial antibody EMA-IgA/IgG. If the tests are positive, then a small intestine biopsy should be done. A positive small intestine biopsy showing damage to the intestinal villi, followed by return of health after adhering to a gluten-free diet, will confirm a diagnosis of celiac disease.[8]

Although gluten is a protein molecule that interacts with T-cell receptors of the immune system to trigger inflammation, physicians in the United States most often help people manage the consequences of (as opposed to preventing) inflammation. This emphasis on treating symptoms typically results in a prescription for medication. Therefore, the average delay in diagnosis for a person with symptoms of celiac disease is 11 years, and on average, a child will visit eight pediatricians before being diagnosed with celiac disease.[8] Celiac disease is the only autoimmune disorder where the trigger, gluten, is known. Remove the trigger and the auto-immune response does not occur.

The only accepted treatment for celiac disease is a gluten-free diet, a diet free of wheat, rye, and barley. Gluten is one of the most common ingredients in processed foods, and is found in everything from soup stock to soy sauce to butterscotch morsels. Therefore, it is important that people with celiac disease read food ingredient labels and be extremely careful when eating food prepared outside the home.

For more comprehensive information about the disease, we recommend the following resources: *Celiac Disease: A Hidden Epidemic* by Dr. Peter Green and Rory Jones (Harper-Collins 2006); the Gluten Intolerance Group of North America website (http://gluten.net); Celiac.com (http://www.celiac.com); and the National Digestive Diseases Information Clearinghouse, a service of the National Institute of Diabetes and Digestive and Kidney Diseases (http://digestive.niddk.nih.gov/).

Nonceliac Gluten Intolerance

Some persons who experience distress when eating gluten-containing products and show improvement after following a gluten-free diet may have nonceliac gluten intolerance instead of celiac disease. Nonceliac gluten intolerance generally worsens over time, but, unlike celiac disease, there may be no damage to the small intestine.[5] Gluten intolerance is caused by a defect in the body's ability to digest the gliadin protein in gluten: humans do not have the proper enzymatic capacity to completely break down the gliadin protein into small digestible molecules. Inflammation occurs and damage to the intestinal wall can cause leaky gut syndrome. People with nonceliac gluten intolerance will have negative TTG and EMA blood tests and negative allergy tests to gluten. Nonceliac gluten intolerance is also a delayed hypersensitivity. Symptoms of this type of food sensitivity include gas, intermittent diarrhea, constipation, irritable bowel syndrome, skin rashes, migraine headaches, arthritis, thyroid problems, neurologic problems, asthma, allergies, sinus infections, and an unproductive cough. As with celiac disease, there are more than 200 symptoms associated with nonceliac gluten intolerance, and almost everyone has a different set of symptoms.

Any person who experiences some type of reaction to gluten is gluten sensitive. Those people who are gluten sensitive and have the genetic markers for celiac disease are gluten intolerant, but not all gluten-intolerant persons have celiac disease. Table AB.1 presents the gluten sensitivity spectrum.

TABLE AB.1: GLUTEN SENSITIVITY SPECTRUM ACCORDING TO REACTION AFTER INGESTING GLUTEN

(+ and − signs refer to antibody blood test results)

Immediate Immune Reaction	Delayed Immune Reaction	Autoimmune Reaction
Wheat IgE (+)	Gliadin IgG (+)	Gliadin IgG (+)
Gliadin IgE +	Gliadin IgA (+)	Gliadin IgA (+)
	TTG IgA/IgG (-)	TTG IgA/IgG (+)
	EMA IgA/IgG (-)	EMA IgA/IgG (+)
Allergy	Non-celiac gluten intolerance	Celiac disease
No intestinal villi damage	No intestinal villi damage	Intestinal villi damage
Gluten-free diet beneficial	Gluten-free diet beneficial	Gluten-free diet beneficial

Wheat or Gluten Allergy

A true wheat or gluten allergy symptom can range from mild discomfort to the potentially life-threatening, and symptoms typically occur within minutes to an hour after eating the offending food. Common symptoms of a wheat or gluten allergy include skin irritations, such as rashes, hives, and eczema, and gastrointestinal symptoms, such as nausea, diarrhea, and vomiting.[9]

CONCLUSION

Unquestionably, it is important to understand the difference between celiac disease, gluten intolerance, and wheat allergy. Celiac disease is not a food allergy; rather, it is an autoimmune disease. Food allergies, including wheat allergy, are conditions that people can grow out of and that do not destroy the body's tissues. This is not the case with celiac disease. Celiac disease is an autoimmune condition that puts the patient at risk for other autoimmune conditions, such as thyroid disease, type 1 diabetes, joint diseases, and liver diseases. Because wheat allergy and nonceliac gluten intolerance are not autoimmune conditions, people who have food allergies and intolerances may not be at increased risk to develop an autoimmune condition over the general population's risk, but they may still suffer physical consequences because of the immune system's inflammatory reaction to gluten.

The American College of Gastroenterology estimates that 95 million Americans have gastrointestinal problems. If 12 million of the 95 million have true food allergies, then 83 million, or approximately one of three Americans, have other food sensitivities and intolerances. Quite literally, the food we eat is making us sick. Currently, there is no cure for food allergies, sensitivities, or intolerances. The only way to manage these conditions is strict avoidance of the offending food or food component.

DEFINITIONS

Antibody: A disease-fighting protein the body develops in response to the presence of an antigen. An antibody binds to an antigen and marks the antigen for destruction by other immune system cells.

Antigen: Any substance that produces an immune response

B-cell: A type of white blood cell best known for producing antibodies.

Human leukocyte antigen: Molecules on the surface of cells that allow the body to distinguish itself from foreign—nonself—substances.

Macrophage: A type of white blood cell that circulates in the blood looking for foreign substances. When it finds foreign antigens, such as bacteria, it engulfs and destroys them.

Neutrophils: Another type of white blood cell that circulates in the blood looking for foreign substances. When it finds foreign antigens, such as bacteria, it engulfs and destroys them.

T-cell: A type of white blood cell that helps to destroy infected cells and coordinate the overall immune response.

APPENDIX B REFERENCES

1. Saulo, A. 2002. "Food Allergy and Other Food Sensitivities." Cooperative Extension Service, College of Tropical Agriculture and Human Resources, University of Hawaii at Manoa. *Food Safety and Technology*, Dec 2002, FST-12.

2. Jabri, B., and S. Guandalini, 2006. "Living Well with Celiac Disease: Celiac Disease Research at the University of Chicago." http://www.celiacdisease.net/assets/documents/ CDCFactSheets_Research_v1.pdf. Accessed August 13, 2009.

3. Green, P., and C. Cellier. 2007. "Medical Progress: Celiac Disease." *New England Journal of Medicine* 357:1731–1743.

4. Fasano, A., I. Berti, T. Gerarduzzi, T. Not, R. Colletti, S. Drago, et al. 2003. "Prevalence of Celiac Disease in at-Risk and Not-at-Risk Groups in the United States: A Large Multi-Center Study." *Gastroenterology* 126:359–61.

5. Gluten Intolerance Group of North America, 2006. "Gluten Sensitivity: Could Gluten Intolerance Make Me Feel Sick?" http://www.gluten.net/downloads/print/ glutenintoeranceflat/pdf. Accessed August 13, 2009.

6. Green, P., and R. Jones. 2006. *Celiac Disease: A Hidden Epidemic*. New York: HarperCollins.

7. Murray, J. 2004. Celiac Disease in the 21st Century. Presentation by Dr. Joseph Murray, Mayo Clinic, to the Montana Celiac Society, August 7, Billings Deaconess Hospital, Billings, Montana.

8. National Institute of Health. 2004. National Institutes of Health Consensus Development Conference Statement: Celiac Disease. http//:consensus.nih.gov/2004/2004CeliacDisease/118html.htm. Accessed August 12, 2009.

9. MayoClinic.com. 2009. Wheat Allergy. Mayoclinic.com/health/wheat-allergy/DSO1002/DSECTION=symptoms. Accessed August 13, 2009.

How Does Gluten Sensitivity Increase Your Risk For Obesity?

Two CATEGORIES OF BLOOD CELLS are found in the body: white and red. White blood cells, or leukocytes, are cells of the immune system. They defend the body against infectious disease and foreign materials. Red blood cells, or erythrocytes, are the most common type of blood cell and are responsible for transporting oxygen and carbon dioxide throughout the body. They attach to oxygen, and when they circulate through a tissue that needs oxygen, they release the oxygen and pick up carbon dioxide to bring it back to the lungs. Lipids (fat), proteins, and carbohydrates are the main constituents of red or white cells.

Gluten sensitivity and increased acidity levels overstimulate the white blood cells, which inflames the body's tissues, causing increased cell membrane permeability. As cell membranes become more porous, white blood cells become more activated, resulting in an increase in oxygen-reactive substances and free radicals. These free radicals steal electrons from lipids (fats) in the red blood cells altering their membrane structure and decreasing their cellular fluidity. Alterations of the size, shape, and diffusion capacity of red blood cells decrease tissue oxygenation. Lower levels of oxygen available in cardiovascular and other organ cells might be part of a pathogenic mechanism responsible for obesity and obesity-related illnesses, such as atherosclerosis and hypertension. In addition, the process by which lipids are oxidized by free radicals causes more inflammation and reduces the body's ability to metabolize glucose resulting in insulin resistance.[1]

Insulin resistance describes the condition by which cells have become less sensitive to the effects of insulin, the hormone secreted by the pancreas to help glucose gain entry to cells where it is turned into energy. If you have insulin resistance, your muscle, fat, and liver cells do not use insulin properly. The pancreas tries to keep up with demand for insulin by releasing even more insulin. Eventually, the pancreas cannot keep up with the body's need for insulin, and excess glucose (energy) builds up in the bloodstream increasing your risk for diabetes and metabolic syndrome X. Insulin stores fat. Too much insulin affects the body's ability to use calories efficiently, and the body stores excess energy as fat, thereby causing obesity.

APPENDIX C REFERENCE

1. Cazzola, R., M. Rondanelli, S. Russo-Volpe, E. Ferrari, and B. Cestaro. 2004. "Decreased Membrane Fluidity and Altered Susceptibility to Peroxidation and Lipid Composition in Overweight and Obese Female Erythrocytes." *Journal of Lipid Research* 45:1846–51.

Understanding Your Immune System

THE IMMUNE SYSTEM is a complex series of responses that protects the body from disease by attacking anything foreign to it. An antigen is any substance that causes the immune system to produce antibodies against it. An antigen may be a foreign substance from the environment, such as food proteins, chemicals, bacteria, viruses, or pollen, that has been ingested, inhaled, or injected into the body. An antigen may also be generated within cells, as a result of normal cell metabolism, or because of viral or intracellular bacterial infection. A third type of antigen is a normal protein or complex of proteins (and sometimes DNA or RNA) that is recognized by the immune system of patients suffering from a specific autoimmune disease. An *antibody* is a disease-fighting protein developed by the body in response to the presence of an antigen.

When you ingest something your immune system doesn't like and perceives as undesirable, it attacks by means of inflammation. *T-cell receptors* (white blood cells that help destroy infected cells and coordinate the overall immune response) interact with antigen protein molecules to recognize self antigens. T-cells mediate the immune response and release a message to the *B-cells* (white blood cells best known for making antibodies) to produce antibodies.

An antibody binds to an antigen and marks the antigen for destruction by other immune system cells. B-cells can only make antibodies when they receive the appropriate command from the T-cell. In some autoimmune diseases, B-cells mistakenly make antibodies against tissues of the body (self antigens) instead of foreign antigens. For example, in multiple sclerosis, the immune system targets self nerve tissues of the central nervous system, causing paralysis.

Other types of white blood cells (such as *macrophages* and *neutrophils*) circulate in the blood and survey the body for foreign substances. When they find foreign antigens, such as bacteria, they engulf and destroy them. The antigens are destroyed by the production of toxic molecules, such as reactive oxygen intermediate molecules. If production of these toxic molecules continues unchecked, not only are the foreign antigens destroyed, but tissue surrounding the macrophages and neutrophils are also destroyed. This build-up of toxic molecules contributes to inflammation.

When inflammation occurs, chemicals from the body's white blood cells are released into the blood or affected tissues in an attempt to rid the body of foreign substances. This release of chemicals increases the blood flow to the area and may result in irritation and redness. Some of the chemicals cause leakage of fluid into the tissues, resulting in swelling, stimulating the nerves, and causing pain. For example, in rheumatoid arthritis, toxic molecules are made by overproductive macrophage and neutrophils cells invading the joints, causing warmth and swelling, and resulting in damage to the joint.

When many antibodies are bound to antigens in the bloodstream, they form a lattice network called an *immune complex*. Immune complexes are harmful when they accumulate and initiate inflammation within small blood vessels that nourish tissues. Immune complexes, immune cells, and inflammatory molecules can block blood flow and ultimately destroy organs, such as the kidney. This can occur in people with lupus.[1]

Following are examples of immune system (or autoimmune) diseases listed by human body system:[1]

- **Gastrointestinal system**: celiac disease, Crohn's disease, and ulcerative colitis.
- **Nervous system**: multiple sclerosis and peripheral neuropathy (numbness and pain).
- **Musculoskeletal system**: rheumatoid arthritis.
- **Skin**: systematic lupus erythematosus, dermatitis, scleroderma, psoriasis, and Sjogren's syndrome.
- **Blood**: type 1 diabetes, pernicious and autoimmune hemolytic anemia, and Wegener's granulomatosis.
- **Endocrine**: thyroid disease, Graves' disease, and Hashimoto's thyroiditis.

The most important factors affecting the immune system are nutritional status (diet), lifestyle (physical activity), the physical environment (toxins and stress), and genetics. Genetics are not easily changed. The immune system today is basically identical to that of our 10,000-year-old ancestors. Our physical environment is also often difficult to change in the short term, as few of us can pick up and leave our home, job, family, and friends to live on a pristine island free of pollutants, toxins, and stress.

Therefore, the only way to immediately affect your immune system is through the food you eat and the amount of physical exercise you get each day. And because 50 percent of the immune system surrounds the gastrointestinal tract, what you ingest daily directly affects your nutritional status, toxin levels in your body (antibiotics and poisonous chemicals), and how well you feel. Physical activity is important for good health, but if you eat a diet that weakens the immune system, you negate the benefits of exercise. Also, when you are ill or in pain, exercise becomes difficult. Therefore, the quickest, simplest, and easiest way to strengthen your immune system is to have a healthy, happy gastrointestinal tract through the consumption of a diet of whole foods, such as vegetables, fruits, beans, nuts, wild fish, and lean meats.

APPENDIX D REFERENCE

1. NIAID (National Institute of Allergy and Infectious Disease). 2007. "Understanding Autoimmune Disease." http://www.wrongdiagnosis.com/artic/understanding_autoimmune_disease_niaid.htm (accessed August 1, 2009).

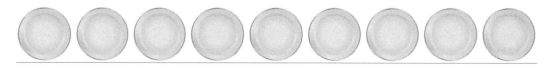

Understanding pH

POTENTIAL OF HYDROGEN, OR pH, is a measure of the acidity or alkalinity of a solution. It is measured on a scale of 0 to 14—the lower the pH the more acidic the solution, the higher the pH the more alkaline (or base) the solution. When a solution is neither acid nor alkaline it has a pH of 7, which is neutral. Following is a list of examples of pH ranging from highly acidic to highly alkaline:

- pH 0: battery acid
- pH 1: hydrochloric acid
- pH 2: lemon juice, vinegar
- pH 3: grapefruit
- pH 4: tomato juice
- pH 5: black coffee
- pH 6: urine, saliva
- pH 7: fresh water, milk
- pH 8: seawater
- pH 9: baking soda
- pH 10: milk of magnesia
- pH 11: ammonia
- pH 12: soap
- pH 13: bleach
- pH 14: liquid drain cleaner

WHY IS pH IMPORTANT?

The human body is able to assimilate minerals and nutrients properly only when its pH is balanced. The human body has a specific pH value, and our bodies continually strive to maintain that specific pH. In fact, each body fluid has a specific pH value. The blood, for example, has a more alkaline pH balance of 7.4. The saliva and urine are more acidic, averaging between 6.5 and 7.0. Optimal balance of the body's pH is necessary to maintain overall health and prevent chronic disease. When this balance is compromised many problems can occur, and your health may also be compromised.

It is important to understand that we are not talking about stomach acid or the pH of the stomach. The stomach needs to be acidic to help digest food. We are talking about the pH of the body's fluids and tissues, which is an entirely different matter. Water makes up 80 percent of the body. Blood is mostly water (82 percent), as are muscles (70 percent) and the brain (85 percent). The human body needs water to regulate body temperature and to provide the means for nutrients to travel to all the organs. Water also transports oxygen to cells, removes waste, and protects the joints and organs. Water is charged with negative ions (called electrons), which function as a potent antioxidant to attract free radicals and to neutralize positively charged toxins (protons) in the blood.

Remember, the human body is composed of many different types of cells, which in turn are composed of many different types of molecules, which consist of one or more atoms of one or more elements joined by chemical bonds. And atoms consist of a nucleus, neutrons, protons, and electrons. Electrons are involved in chemical reactions and are the substance that bonds atoms together to form molecules. The most important structural feature of an atom for determining its chemical behavior is the number of electrons in its outer shell. A substance that has a full outer shell tends not to enter in chemical reactions. By nature, atoms seek stability, so they will try to fill their outer shell by gaining or losing electrons, or sharing electrons by bonding together with other atoms.

When weak bonds split, free radicals are formed. Free radicals are highly charged unstable molecular fragments that may puncture cell membranes, destroy enzymes, and even break down DNA just to steal an electron from another molecule. Some free radicals occur naturally as cells burn food for energy (a process called oxidative metabolism). Other free radicals come from exposure to ultraviolet radiation (sunlight), radon, X-rays, pollutants, pesticides, food additives, alcohol, and other toxins. Sometimes the cells in the body's immune system purposefully create free radicals to neutralize viruses and bacteria.

Generally, free radicals attack the nearest stable molecule, stealing an electron. When the attacked molecule losses its electron, it becomes a free radical itself, beginning a chain reaction that is disruptive to living cells. To give you an idea of how much damage free radicals can do, consider that these renegade molecules strike and fracture every single one of your DNA molecules 10,000 times a day. About 9,900 of these breaks in the DNA strand are restored to normal by DNA repair enzymes. About 100, or 1 percent, escape the enzymes' notice. This damage accumulates over time, setting the stage for atherosclerosis, cancer, and other degenerative diseases.[1]

Overacidity of fluids in the body due to diet[2] reduces the potent antioxidant function of water, thereby weakening all body systems. A healthy body maintains adequate alkaline re-serves to meet emergency demands. When excess acids must be neutralized, alkaline reserves are depleted, leaving the body in a weakened condition. To counteract the cellular problems caused by mild acidity, the body's innate mechanism of self-regulation draws on its alkali mineral stores of calcium, magnesium, and potassium within the musculoskeletal system. Consistent mineral withdrawal can lead to osteoporosis (a common bone disease that occurs from the thinning of bone tissue and loss of bone density over time), spinal degeneration, tooth decay, dry skin and nails, and rheumatism.[3] A pH-neutral diet is vital to the strength and maintenance of the musculoskeletal system.

Cellular problems also lead to premature aging of cells because the body's organs become weakened from mineral withdrawal. In the brain, impaired mental acuity and memory prob-lems can result, contributing to dementia and early Alzheimer's disease.

Over time, even mild acidity in the body can cause such problems as

- Weakened immune system, increased stress, and higher blood pressure
- Gastrointestinal disorders, such as diarrhea, constipation, bloating, and gas
- Cardiovascular damage, including blood vessel constriction, clogged arteries, weak-ened veins, and the reduction of oxygen
- All forms of cancer
- Unwanted weight/fat gain and obesity
- Insulin disorders and diabetes
- Liver, bladder, and kidney conditions, including kidney stones and gallstones
- Neurologic diseases, such as multiple sclerosis, Lou Gehrig's disease (amyotrophic lateral sclerosis), Parkinson's disease, and Alzheimer's disease
- Premature aging, frequent headaches, sinusitis, and hemorrhoids
- Osteoporosis, weak or brittle bones, hip fractures, bone spurs, and calcium deposits
- Osteoarthritis, joint pain, aching muscles, and lactic acid buildup
- Hormonal imbalances, prostate problems, and adult acne
- Low energy, chronic fatigue, and fibromyalgia

HOW DOES FRESH LEMON JUICE NEUTRALIZE ACIDITY IN THE BODY?

Fresh lemon juice is highly stable, is water soluble, and contains a negatively charged ion. Negative charges (electrons) attract positive charges (protons). Therefore, lemon juice provides the electrons to neutralize free radicals in blood and help to prevent cell and tissue damage that could lead to cellular damage and disease. After they lose electrons, lemon juice molecules do not become free radicals because they are highly stable antioxidants, with or without the electrons. Lemon juice increases the potent antioxidant function of water in our body.

APPENDIX E REFERENCES

1. Ozawa, T. 1999. *Understanding the Process of Aging.* New York: Marcel Dekker, 265–292.

2. Frassetto L., R. Morris, D. Sellmeyer, and A. Sebastian. 2008. "Adverse Effects of Sodium Chloride on Bone in the Aging Human Population Resulting from Habitual Consumption of Typical American Diets." *Journal of Nutrition* 138:419–22.

3. Bobkov, V.A., T.N. Brylenkova, E.I. Kopilov, S.G. Mitskaia, N.I. Kazakova. 1999. "Changes in the Acid-Base Status of the Synovial Fluid in Rheumatoid Arthritis Patients." *Terapevticheski Arkhiv* (Russia) 71(5):20–2.

Gluten-Free Baking

Excerpted from Gluten-Free Baking Classics, Second Edition, by Annalise Roberts

IF YOU THINK ABOUT HOW MOST PEOPLE BAKE WITH WHEAT, you will realize that they usually use two different kinds of flour: an all-purpose flour for cakes, pies, muffins, and other pastries, and a bread flour for baking bread. The recipes in this book use just two flour mixes: the Brown Rice Flour Mix (my all-purpose flour) makes cakes, pies, muffins and cookies that look, feel, and taste like those made with wheat, and the Bread Flour Mix (my bread flour) makes crusty, chewy artisan loaves and tender sandwich breads.

THE SCIENCE OF BAKING WITH GLUTEN-FREE FLOURS

Few people I know have large amounts of time to bake, much less to grab for four different flours each time they do. Fewer still have room to store three or four different flour mixes in their cabinets. Following my philosophy that cooking should be simple, I want to be able to reach for a gluten-free all-purpose flour or a gluten-free bread flour and know it will work dependably for everything I make. The recipes in this book are carefully calibrated to work with the flour combinations given below. Be aware that if you do in fact substitute flours, it will probably be necessary to adjust the amounts of other ingredients you use (most likely xanthan gum, liquids, and leavening agents).

Gluten-Free All-Purpose Flour for Cakes, Pies, Muffins, and Cookies

My "all-purpose" Brown Rice Flour Mix is a combination of extra finely ground brown rice flour, potato starch (not potato flour), and tapioca flour (also called tapioca starch).

Food Philosopher Gluten-Free Brown Rice Flour Mix

Brown rice flour (extra finely ground)	2 parts	2 cups	6 cups
Potato starch (not potato flour)	⅔ part	⅔ cup	2 cups
Tapioca flour	⅓ part	⅓ cup	1 cup
Total		**3 cups**	**9 cups**

It is very important that you use an extra finely ground brown rice flour (not just any grind), or your baked goods will be gritty, heavy and/or crumbly. At this time, Authentic Foods in California sells the only one I can find other than those sold in Asian grocery stores. Authentic Foods rice flour is powdery, just like all-purpose wheat flour. It can be bought online and in natural food stores; the mailing address, email address, and phone number can be found at the end of this chapter. Take note: Authentic Foods now makes the above Brown Rice Flour Mix already made up under the name GF Classic Blend.

The other brands of brown rice flour have a larger grind that you can actually feel between your fingers. They are not powdery (as of this writing), and it really does make a difference. If you want or need to use one of these other brands, try to find one with the finest grind you can. Buy several at a time, if you can. Open the packages and feel the flour. Use the finest grinds for cakes, muffins, cookies, and pie crusts. Use the coarser grinds for pizza.

The potato starch and tapioca flour can be found in local natural food stores, some grocery stores, and online. The brands seem fairly interchangeable and are consistent in quality.

In addition to the Brown Rice Flour Mix above, the pie crust recipe calls for sweet rice flour, which helps give certain baked goods a better texture. Only a small amount is ever used at a time, because too much results in a denser, tighter, and gummy product. It is available in local natural food stores, some grocery stores, and online. I recommend extra finely ground Authentic Foods sweet rice flour, or your crust will be gritty.

Gluten-Free Flours for Bread

If you are like me, you have baked and eaten more than your fair share of bad gluten-free bread. Over time, I developed recipes and a flour mix for making some of the breads I missed most. It will allow you to make breads that taste good, rise evenly, and won't fall when they come out of the oven. If you follow the detailed instructions, your gluten-free yeast breads will have the "mouth feel" and texture of the wheat breads you are familiar with. Moreover, they do not contain rice flour, so they will not have the gummy, glossy look and feel of many of the gluten-free breads you see in stores or ones that you may have baked in the past.

My bread flour mix is made up of whole-grain flours and starch flours in a ratio of half to half; a combination of millet, sorghum, corn starch, potato starch (not potato flour), and tapioca flour (also called tapioca starch). Millet and sorghum are used to help vary the taste, improve nutrition, and provide structure to the dough. The starches help lighten the texture and improve mouth feel.

Bread Flour Mix A uses more millet than sorghum and has a very slight golden hue and makes a sandwich bread that is much like homemade wheat bread in terms of texture and density. The millet and sorghum flour (both whole grain) help keep the loaves fresher than gluten-free breads made of all starchy flours. But, remember that real homemade wheat breads never have a shelf life as long as the commercially produced loaves sold in grocery stores today, and neither will your homemade gluten-free bread.

Food Philosopher Gluten-Free Bread Flour Mix

⅓ part millet flour	2 cups	⅔ cup	½ cup
⅙ part sorghum flour	1 cup	⅓ cup	¼ cup
⅙ part cornstarch	1 cup	⅓ cup	¼ cup
⅙ part potato starch	1 cup	⅓ cup	¼ cup
⅙ part tapioca flour	1 cup	⅓ cup	¼ cup
Total	**6 cups**	**2 cups**	**1½ cups**

The millet, sorghum, potato starch, tapioca flour, and "gluten-free" oatmeal can be found in local natural food stores, some grocery stores, and online. The brands seem fairly interchangeable and are consistent in quality. Corn starch can be found in any grocery store.

GLUTEN-FREE FLOURS FOR PIZZA

The pizza recipe in this book uses the Brown Rice Flour Mix but does not require finely ground brown rice flour. It will actually have an improved texture if made with a coarser-ground flour. Although I usually use my regular Brown Rice Flour Mix above, I will go out of my way to buy brown rice flour with a coarser grind when I know I'm going to bake a lot of pizza crusts for the freezer. Bob's Red Mill brown rice flour is great for pizza crust, and I am lucky enough to find it at my local grocery store. It can also be found in local natural food stores or ordered online. But there are many other brands of coarser ground brown rice flour, so you will no doubt be able to find one you like. In addition to the Brown Rice Flour Mix, I use millet flour in pizza, although the recipe can be made without it (just substitute more of the brown rice flour). I think millet adds a bit of complexity to the texture and taste, and I like to use it whenever I make pizza.

HOW TO MEASURE AND MIX GLUTEN-FREE FLOURS

To measure flour for making flour mixes: Put the empty measuring cup into a small bowl. Use a soup spoon to spoon the flour from the package into the measuring cup, or pour the flour from the package into the measuring cup. Then use a knife or spoon handle to level the top (do this over the bowl to avoid a messy cleanup; pour the flour left in the bowl back into the package or another container). Do not scoop gluten-free flours directly out of the package with the measuring cup.

As each flour is measured, transfer it into a plastic container large enough to leave four or five inches from the top unfilled. Shake container vigorously to mix flours. I usually make 12 cups of Brown Rice Flour Mix at a time and store and shake it in a 21-cup Rubbermaid container.

To measure flour for use in recipes: Shake storage container vigorously to mix and aerate the flour mix. Put the empty measuring cup into a small bowl, or hold it over the opening of the container if it is large enough. Use a soup spoon to spoon the flour from the container into the measuring cup, then use a knife or spoon handle to level the top. If you do this over a bowl, pour the flour left in the bowl back into the storage container. Do not scoop gluten-free flours out of the storage container with the measuring cup. Remember: Shake and bake!

HOW TO PURCHASE AND STORE GLUTEN-FREE FLOURS

Brown rice flour, millet flour, and sorghum, are whole-grain flours and must be stored carefully. The Brown Rice Flour Mix and the Bread Flour Mix can be stored at room temperature for about four months. If your house is hot and humid, or if you will not be baking for long periods of time, store the mixes in the refrigerator. Store open packages of brown rice flour, millet flour, and sorghum in the refrigerator.

Purchase all these flours from stores or online sellers that have a lot of turnover, so you can be sure you are getting fresh packages. Do not purchase them too far in advance of when you make the flour mixes (more than four months). When you open a new bag, make sure it does not have a strong odor, an indication that it is rancid or old. These flours should have a pleasant, grainy, nutty smell. Millet flour in particular tends to get rancid if not stored properly or if it is old (just like whole-wheat flour). Old flours often impart a bitter taste in your baked goods.

Both open and unopened packages of potato starch, tapioca flour, and corn starch can be stored at room temperature for more than a year. They can be purchased in advance of when you will be using them to make the flour mixes.

INDEX

L

Lamb
    Grilled Tandoori Lamb with Cucumber Raita, 253–254
    Moroccan Lamb Stew, 251–252
    Roasted Leg of Lamb with Garlic Crust, 250
Leaky gut syndrome, 28–29
Lemon Soufflé, 263
Lemons, alkalinity and, 42, 285
Lentils
    Dal (Curried Lentils), 121
    Lentil Soup, 106–107
Lunch suggestions, 41, 54, 57–59

M

Magnesium, sources of, 46
Manhattan Clam Chowder, 119–120
Marinades, 74–75
Mashed Potatoes, 145
Meats, art and science of purchasing, 211–212. *See also* Beef; Buffalo; Lamb; Pork; Veal
Mediterranean Lunch Plate, 59
Mexican Chicken Tortilla Casserole, 218
Milk substitutes, 75
Minerals, sources of, 46
Moroccan Lamb Stew, 251–252
Mousse, Chocolate, 267
Mozzarella cheese
    Chicken Parmesan, 223–224
    Tomato, Mozzarella, and Grilled Red Onion Salad, 159
Muffins, gluten-free flours for, 286–287
Mushrooms
    Asian-Style Grilled Vegetable Platter, 142–143
    Beef Stir-Fry with Oyster Sauce, 233
    Beef Stroganoff, 231–232
    Chicken Marsala, 214–215
    Creamy Mushroom Garlic Sauce Base, 89
    Creamy Mushroom Sauce Base for Gravy and Soup, 88
    Creamy Mushroom Soup, 114
    Green Beans with Shiitake Mushrooms, 155

    Old-Fashioned Saucepan Mushroom Gravy, 95
    Pasta with Creamy Gorgonzola and Mushroom Sauce, 173
Mussels, Steamed, 200

N

Nectarines, Poached, 262
Nonceliac gluten intolerance, 273

O

Oats, in Sesame Oatmeal Rolls, 187–188
Obesity, gluten sensitivity and, 277–278
Okra, Roasted, 133
Old-fashioned saucepan gravies
    Beef, 94
    Chicken, 93
    Mushroom, 95
Olives
    Kale with Puttanesca Sauce, 157
    Thyme-Scented Green Olives, 165
    Tomato, Caper, and Olive Tapenade, 203
Omega-3 fats, 47
Oven-Fried Sweet Potatoes, 137

P

Pancakes, Buckwheat, 189–190
Pancetta, in Bean Pot Base, 102–103
Parsnips, in Roasted Winter Vegetable Soup, 112–113
Pasta
    Chicken Noodle Gratin, 169–170
    Macaroni and Cheese, 176–177
    Pasta with Chicken and Creamy Pesto Sauce, 174–175
    Pasta with Creamy Gorgonzola and Mushroom Sauce, 173
    Pasta with Spicy Ratatouille and Goat Cheese, 139
Pastes, 75

ABOUT THE AUTHORS

After being diagnosed with celiac disease in 2002, Annalise Roberts devoted herself to developing gluten-free baking recipes that taste just as good (if not better than) their wheat flour counterparts. Her recipes were featured in *Gourmet* magazine in November 2005, and her first book, *Gluten-Free Baking Classics* (Agate Surrey) appeared in May 2006 (an expanded and revised edition was released in September 2008). Her most recent book, *Gluten-Free Baking Classics for the Bread Machine* (Agate Surrey, 2009), is a collection of recipes developed for the Zojirushi bread machine. She works with celiac support groups and teaches gluten-free cooking and baking classes in the New York–New Jersey metropolitan area, and produces and manages the Web site www.foodphilosopher.com with her sister, Claudia.

In 2007, Claudia Pillow received her Ph.D. in Health Studies from Texas Women's University but she has been studying and working with food for her entire life. Dr. Pillow is a classically trained chef and graduate of the New York Restaurant School, and she worked as a chef and caterer for many years in the New York metropolitan area. An MBA offered her the opportunity to jump to the corporate side of the food industry, where she marketed cheese and natural beverages. Currently, she lectures about gluten intolerance and teaches gluten-free cooking and baking classes in the Dallas/Fort Worth area. Dr. Pillow serves on the board of the Gluten Intolerance Group of North America and is a local resource for the North Texas chapter. Together with her sister, Annalise, she manages and produces the Web site www.foodphilosopher.com.